Overcoming Asthma and Hay Fever

Proven drug-free methods to combat the causes

Note to reader

Before following the self-help advice given in this book readers are earnestly urged to give careful consideration to the nature of their particular health problem, and to consult a competent physician if in any doubt.

This book should not be regarded as a substitute for professional medical treatment, and whilst every care is taken to ensure the accuracy of the content, the author and the publishers cannot accept legal responsibility for any problem arising out of the experimentation with the methods described.

Contents

1. Common factors in asthma and hay fever

There are two major reasons for grouping these two quite separate conditions together. These are that both have roots in allergic reactions, and both to a large degree involve the respiratory organs of the body. To the extent that there are common factors, there are also similarities in the methods which are available for self-help, both in coping with these conditions, and in attempting to achieve freedom from their periodic recurrence. It is also well established that a high proportion (between 30 and 40 per cent) of children who are hay fever sufferers will develop asthma.

In order to understand the reasons for some of the methods of self-help which will be outlined in later chapters, it is necessary, from the outset, to understand something of the mechanics of allergic reactions.

In order to do this we must look at the major defence system of the body, the immune system, and the manner in which this can become oversensitive, or over-reactive. We should also examine, to some extent, the mechanisms involved in the body which are affected by these particular allergic manifestations.

To simply label a condition as 'allergic' does not gain us very much if we fail to understand the many factors which can be involved in such a process. The allergic reaction is the last event in a chain of incidents of great complexity. The fact that someone is sensitive to, or allergic to, a particular substance - whether this be a food, a pollen, a chemical, or any other substance - does not explain the problem; it only identifies the existence of that particular sensitivity. Avoidance of the substance does not, in itself, achieve very much in the long term, but gains only a respite from current symptoms. The underlying dysfunction of the immune system remains, and can be manifested in a return of symptoms, in response to other substances or circumstances, if nothing is done to correct the basic problem.

In all human ill health there are seldom simple causes. Few conditions have only a single cause: rather, there are multi-factorial influences at work.

These include inherited tendencies (all too common a factor in allergic problems) as well as nutritional imbalances, stress factors, emotional or psychological elements, etc. There is also strong evidence to support the view of osteopathic and chiropractic practitioners that there is frequently a structural, or mechanical, element present (especially in the case of asthma) which predisposes the individual to that particular expression of disease or dysfunction.

Thus, with many interacting elements involved in the way a condition such as asthma or hay fever becomes active, we need to look at some of the background events in order to see just what we can do to prevent, and to ease, the condition. We should also look at the current medical therapies used to treat these conditions, and assess their suitability, desirability, side-effects, etc.

It is worth emphasizing that the enormous attention that allergy in general has attracted from the healing professions, over the past few years, has gained us a greater insight into those phenomena which closely mimic true allergy. Thus it is now common to hear conditions described as 'sensitivities', rather than allergies;' the difference between these two words, or descriptions, is quite important, as we will discover.

I will now explain just what happens in the body when an allergy is involved.

2. Allergy and sensitivity

When a substance which the body believes to be dangerous enters the body, by any route (it may be eaten, breathed or taken in through the skin), defence mechanisms begin to operate to deal with this challenge.

This is happening all the time, in the body's unobserved effort to maintain a balanced, safe, harmonious, inner environment. When such efforts become exaggerated, and begin to operate against substances which may or may not be a threat to the body, we label the condition as an allergy. This, as we shall see, can happen for a number of reasons.

The normalizing and balancing mechanism in the body is called its 'homoeostatic' mechanism. This can be alerted by the presence in the system of substances which have been inadequately dealt with by the digestive system, and which have entered the bloodstream in this partially digested form. This often happens when an infant has been fed foods with which the digestive system is not yet sufficiently developed to cope. Alternatively, damage to the digestive capabilities, at any age, can result in inadequate protein breakdown (for example when pancreatic function is weak and enzyme production is insufficient). Also, if, through infection and chronic irritation; the wall of the bowel becomes inefficient in its ability to allow through to the bloodstream only those substances which it should, then there is another reason for the presence of undesirable substances in the bloodstream, and of a consequent defensive reaction, or over-reaction, by the homoeostatic mechanism.

As already mentioned, such substances can also enter the body via the skin, (injection, bite, etc.), or the lungs. The immediate response is for signals to be sent for antibodies to attack and neutralize any such 'foreign' substance. This is normal, essential, and desirable. We would not live for very long if our bodies did not have this ability.

Histamine

If antibodies attack a 'foreign' protein that has entered the bloodstream, or body, one of the results is the production of a substance called histamine. This is toxic, and among other effects produces swelling and inflammation. If such a reaction took place in the mucous membrane of the lungs then breathing would become difficult and the result might be wheezing or asthma. Normally the body produces its remedy for the presence of histamine, and not surprisingly this is called antihistamine. When healthy, our livers produce this, and the toxic histamine, resulting from the body attacking the undesirable alien substance, is neutralized.

If, however, the body is absorbing a vast number of molecules to which it is reacting in this way or if its enzyme production is faulty through pancreatic dysfunction, or if the liver is unable to produce enough antihistamine, then an allergic condition results.

This simple picture becomes more complicated when we incorporate the effects of emotional stress. It has been clearly established that allergies can produce emotional and psychological effects. Such stresses can themselves contribute to allergic reactions. When aroused by a stimulus, whether through an irritation such as being stuck in a traffic jam on the way to an important meeting, or a defensive reaction, such as happens when the house is on fire, or a long-term worry such as unemployment, changes occur in the body to prepare it for activity. In the case of the house fire, the 'fight or flight' preparation of the body is followed by appropriate activity - running for your life in this case. This uses up the adrenaline and other hormones which have been produced in response to the initial stimulus. If there is a constant arousal of this sort (anxiety, stressful job, deadlines to meet) and there is no tension release, or adequate response, then there is a tendency for the adrenal glands to eventually become exhausted, and to produce inadequate adrenaline.

One effect of this is a breakdown of the homoeostatic mechanism, with a failure to deal with environmental changes such as temperature alterations, or an inability to maintain normal blood sugar levels, and an increase in sensitivity to otherwise well-tolerated foods and substances. If, through chronic stress we become sensitive too or allergic too, commonly eaten foods, (or commonly breathed substances such as petrol fumes), then the consequent symptoms can be seen to relate primarily to the initial stress factor, and only secondly to the irritant or food.

Where allergy results from the inability of the body to adequately digest a food, for instance milk, then it is logical, as a first step, to stop drinking milk. If, however, the cause lies in either-a pancreatic dysfunction (producing inadequate protein-digesting enzymes) or a toxic liver (unable to detoxify the histamine produced by antibody activity), then, if possible, these organs must be detoxified and normalized. To simply stop the intake of the food to which the body is reacting is not a cure, but an evasive, stop-gap action.

If there is an absorption problem, resulting from the too early introduction to the infant of certain foods, then such evasive action may be all that is possible. If, though, the cause of the allergic symptoms lies in emotional and environmental stress, then these must be the main areas to which therapeutic efforts are directed.

Multiple causes

It is now clear that allergies do not have just one cause. The outline I have given of possible causes does not include all the permutations of factors that can result in an allergic condition. Among the others are a breakdown in the body's ability to handle sugar, due to excessive refined sugar intake, and consequent blood sugar irregularities; spinal dysfunction resulting in over-stimulation of adrenal and pancreatic activity, through over-reaction of the nerves that supply them and consequent allergic symptoms; mineral and vitamin imbalances, due to nutritionally inadequate dietary patterns, which result in the homoeostatic ability of the body becoming impaired, etc.

Since there are so many possible causes, and since, in any individual several of these causes may be operating at the same time (e.g. adrenal exhaustion, toxic liver, and some degree of emotional stress) there is no simple solution to the problem.

Parents must take responsibility for not introducing food to a child before the digestive apparatus (enzyme production) is capable of coping with its proper digestion. This means that, if at all possible, breastfeeding is a must, and this should provide all the nutriment for the first six months.

Most allergies that start in the early months of a person's life relate to cow's milk and cereal products, and these should play no part in the child's diet before six months. At the very first sign of a food not being well-tolerated (colic, restlessness, vomiting, diarrhoea, rashes) that particular food should be stopped.

I should like to stress my convictions that cow's milk has little to commend it as a human food, and that it seems to be related to many problems like arthritis, catarrh, colitis, and allergy. The undesirable effects of dairy products keep cropping up in such conditions.

If either parent has an allergy history then particular care needs to be taken regarding these early stages of feeding. In my experience a vegetarian mode of feeding, using an abundance of fresh fruits and cooked or raw vegetables, together with the judicious use of whole cereals and pulses, provides the safest introduction to solid eating for the child. The longer that supplemental breastfeeding can continue the better. Allergies are rare among breastfed, whole food and vegetarian children.

However, once allergy has manifested itself, whether in a child or in an adult, it is necessary to tackle causes and not symptoms, and one such symptom is the sensitivity or allergy itself. Avoidance of the irritant food or substance is desirable in the short-term, but it does nothing to correct the dysfunction of the organ or systems which is resulting in allergy. This is why I question the long-term validity of focusing attention on tracking down the particular substances to which the person is allergic, unless at the same time something constructive is being done about the underlying causes.

Total holistic therapy takes into account all elements in this complex picture. To concentrate on only one aspect is to court disappointment. To concentrate on the symptoms alone is to court disaster. The various methods that are employed to pinpoint specific substances and foods to which the individual is allergic should be seen as a starting point. Having identified items, the next task is to rebuild the body so that it will no longer react to these substances in an aberrant manner. A healthy body will not produce an allergic reaction.

The mechanisms involved

In order to understand what is, and what is not, an allergic reaction, we must look for a moment at the mechanisms involved it! the reaction. This is a vastly complicated area of study, and it is necessary to simplify the complexities in order to gain some overall awareness of the processes involved, without getting bogged down in the minutiae of the biochemistry.'

When there is an adverse reaction to a food, or some other factor (inhaled or injected substance for example), there can -be one of two general classifications as to what is happening.

There might be a true immunological reaction (allergy), in which case the substance involved would have provoked what is called an antibody reaction.

When a foreign or undesirable substance (or bacteria or virus) enters the system, the defence mechanism may regard this as an allergen or antigen, and a specific antibody will attempt to neutralize this. The antibody, or defence agent, is often in such instances a particular serum protein called an immunoglobulin (Ig). There are a number of different forms of this immunoglobulin (1g), but the one involved in most food allergies, and hay fever, is called immunoglobulin-E (IgE).

If on the other hand there is an intolerance to a particular food substance, which is not truly allergic, then it would not involve the immune system, and there would be no defence by IgE, or other similar factors, involved in such processes. Rather there could be actual toxic, or poisonous, effects, resulting from certain ingested or inhaled substances. Many different reactions can occur in the body as a result of such toxic factors (food poisoning is one such effect) and a variety of symptom patterns can emerge.

Hay fever and asthma almost always involve true immune reactions, with the mediation of antibodies such as IgE. Most of the signs and symptoms of food allergy involve the skin (hives, itching, eczema, etc.), the respiratory system, (sneezing, wheezing, etc.), the cardiovascular system (palpitations, collapse, etc.) or the eyes (redness and watering, and extreme sensitivity). It is now also known that so called 'brain allergies' may result. In such cases anxiety, depression and many varied emotional and psychological manifestations are responsible. There is also known to be an allergic state in which the joints and muscles of the body are disturbed by symptoms which can include arthritis, muscle and joint pain, stiffness, fatigue, etc.

Hay fever is a seasonal condition which can arise very suddenly, and is characterized by a swelling of the mucous lining of the nasal passages, leading to hyper secretion of liquid, and which involves the eyes, leaving them watering and sensitive to light. There is a generalized inflammation of the whole of the upper respiratory tract. The seasonal pattern of the condition implicates spores or pollen, and thus can be related to either the autumn or spring seasons. If mould spores are involved then there is a good chance that there is an involvement in the system of fungal infection, such as Candida albicans. This will be considered in a later chapter. Approximately 30 to 40 per cent of individuals who develop hay fever will, at some stage, also develop symptoms of bronchial asthma.

The nature of asthma is of spasm of the bronchi, and a paroxysmal cough with the presence of noisy wheezing on breathing out. The whole breathing process becomes extremely difficult, but the most characteristic feature of asthma is the difficulty attached to breathing out. Thus air becomes trapped in the bronchioles, and this makes the subsequent inhalation difficult. This pattern of breathing results in inadequate oxygen intake, placing a strain on the heart and circulatory functions. It also fails to allow clearance of acidic wastes from the system (a major element in the function of breathing) and a generalized increase in body acidity results. Secretions in the lungs can become viscous, and further complicate the breathing pattern, making coughing a tiresome complication of the difficulty in breathing.

The terror of the situation, especially in children, adds to the problems, as muscular tensions and contractions further mitigate against adequate breathing.

There are other possible reasons for the presence of asthma, but allergy is the major cause. These others can include cardiac disease, as well as other diseases of the lungs. However, in this book I shall concentrate on the major form of asthma; that which derives from an allergic condition. Asthmatic attacks, in a sensitive individual, can be triggered by almost any stress factor (once the condition exists), such as change of temperature, emotional disturbance, pollution in the atmosphere, exertion, overeating, etc.

Self-help approach

The self-help approach to the problems of hay fever and asthma focuses on improving the ability of the body to deal with the allergens involved, and detoxification, in order to improve the function of those organs and systems which are most involved in the pattern of allergy causation (such as the digestive organs, liver, pancreas, circulatory and lymphatic systems, etc.) The organs most involved in the respiratory function of the body also deserve attention.

The methods that can be used are varied, and include nutritional adjustments; supplementation of nutrients; detoxification via fasting and specific forms of hydrotherapy; exercises and breathing methods; relaxation, meditation and other stress reducing methods; introduction of ionized air; acupressure methods; and the use of safe natural medication, derived from herbal and homoeopathic methods, for symptomatic relief.

The use of medical drug methods in the control of asthma should not be stopped without consultation with a qualified practitioner, such as a clinical ecologist (specialist in allergy), a naturopathic practitioner (specializing in nutritional and non-drug therapies) a homoeopathic practitioner, or a doctor sympathetic to a non-drug approach. It would be potentially dangerous to simply drop drug therapy, and switch to an approach such as the one advocated in this book. This is not to say that it is not possible to achieve a control of such a condition without the use of drugs, but that precipitous change to such an approach is unwise.

Drugless control should be a major objective, but the time scale to achieve this may involve many months.

Before considering self-help, we will briefly look at the current medical approach to the problems of hay fever and asthma.

3. Medical methods and their consequences

The ever vigilant defence mechanisms of the body respond to infecting micro-organisms by attempting to neutralize them. The microbe, virus, etc. (also known as the antigen) will call into action the antibody appropriate to its particular construction, and the body will use this antibody (globulin) to prevent further incursion of the foreign (to it) protein. When this type of action occurs, not in response to microorganisms but in regard to exposure to substances to which the body has become sensitized, such as pollen, dust, animal-hairs, spores, chemicals, etc., we have an allergic reaction, in which the defence mechanism is inappropriately involved. Since all people are exposed to some such potential irritants, and far from all respond in this way, it must be seen as an aberrant over-reaction. The reasons for this have been touched on in the previous chapter, and our present task is to see just how medical science proposes to stop this happening, and why natural self-help measures are frequently superior.

The main- feature of the initial allergic reaction is that there is a release into the system of a substance called histamine (as well as a number of the other substances). The effect of this is to invoke an alarm reaction in which, depending upon the tissues or organs involved, a wide variety of symptoms can be displayed. If the contact with the allergen is through an inhaled substance, such as pollen, then the alarm reaction would be noted in the lining of the respiratory apparatus. Initially this means the nose, sinuses, eyes and upper respiratory channels. Such reactions can be violent or mild, long-lasting or transient, local or widespread, and in some cases can be so serious as to threaten life itself.

Histamine is present in most body tissues, and when a cell is injured it is released. The immediate effect is to open or dilate the local blood vessels, giving a flushed appearance to the tissues involved as blood fills these small vessels. The walls of these blood vessels are made more permeable by the action of histamine, and this leads to the seeping into the surrounding tissues of fluid (plasma). The result of this is swollen tissues (called oedema).

A number of other things happen, almost simultaneously when histamine is released in response to injury, or to the introduction of an allergen. Apart from the local reaction, the blood vessels in the brain may also become dilated, and this can result in headache. To meet the demand of the dilated blood vessels there is often an increase in heart rate, and there is almost always a drop in the blood pressure. If the reaction is particularly severe, this can lead to collapse, and even death. One of the consequences of a histamine release is to contact the narrow tubules in the lungs (bronchioles) and this can lead to asthmatic breathing. The stomach response to histamine is to increase acid production. It has been noted, over the years, that not all the many reactions found in allergies are the result of histamine release, but it is certainly a major factor in many allergies.

The emotional factor

Not only physical factors need to be present in order to trigger a histamine response. Most of us are aware of the itching irritation caused by contact with stinging nettles.

This plant contains histamine, and the nettle rash that results from contact with it is a pure histamine reaction. Many people develop nettle-rash (urticaria) in response to emotional stress, and this should indicate to us just how important is the need for a lack of emotional disturbance, or stress, in anyone subject to allergic reactions. This aspect of the self-help programme will be dealt with in a later chapter on stress reduction. This should not be thought of as merely peripheral to the problem, but something that lies at its very heart.

Of the drugs used in dealing with immediate allergic reactions, the antihistamines are probably the best known. They have their effect, not by stopping the production of histamine but rather, by actually occupying the binding sites in the tissues that histamine would use. They are not totally effective in this role, however, and would best be seen as substances which antagonize the effect of histamine, and not as counteracting all its effects. Antihistamines tend to block histamine's action in the bronchial tubes, and they reduce the degree of skin reaction noted. They are also effective in reducing the symptoms of hay fever. If this were all they did they might be seen as an acceptable form of symptom relief. Unfortunately, since they are attacking a symptom and not a cause (allergy is not caused by histamine, it is merely an expression of the allergic reaction) they have a predictable number of side-effects. Usually they have a depressing effect on the brain (rarely, a stimulating effect is noted). This results in drowsiness and a desire for sleep. When large doses are used, convulsions may result.

According to a noted specialist in the field of the pharmacological effects of drugs, Professor Peter Parish (author of *Medicines: a Guide for Everybody,* Penguin 1987) the reaction to the use of antihistamines varies widely. He states quite directly, 'In effective dosage *all antihistamines* produce adverse effects'.

Among those listed are drowsiness, dizziness, head noises, lack of co-ordination, fatigue, blurred vision, double vision, mood changes, delusions, hallucinations, insomnia, tremors, nausea, loss of appetite, vomiting, dry mouth, constipation or diarrhoea, urinary frequency or difficulty in passing urine, cough, palpitation, tightness of the chest, headache, tingling and weakness of the hands, etc.

Antihistamine

It is also possible to become allergic to antihistamine, especially when its application is to the skin. As far as hay fever is concerned the use of antihistamines is generally found to be of benefit in dealing with the symptoms, but to have no effect whatever on the causes. Since a large proportion of hay fever sufferers eventually become asthmatic, it is vital that causes be dealt with, and that the approach is not confined to symptomatic relief alone. Antihistamines are quite useless in the treatment of asthma.

The use of antihistamines, in some children, can have quite alarming consequences, and there have been reports of birth defects in children of women using these drugs during pregnancy. Their use should be severely restricted to the short-term, if they are felt to be absolutely essential.

The other main medical approach to the problem of hay fever is the use of desensitizing injections. This calls for specific identification of the substance(s) involved in the allergy, which is itself not an easy task, as many people have multiple allergies, and in some cases these change all the time. Once identified, a series of injections, containing minute amounts of the substances involved, are given under the skin, until the body develops a degree of tolerance to them. This method mayor may not be effective, and can require many months of regular injections each year. It also does nothing to correct the causes of the problem, and so leaves the field wide open for other substances to create similar sensitivity problems.

It can be seen from the above that the use of medical methods to deal with hay fever is restricted to symptom obliteration, and not to finding (let alone dealing with) the cause of the problem. The self-help methods which are outlined will attempt to address causes, where possible.

In looking at the drug approach to asthma it is vital to stress that whilst this fails to address causes, it is at times life-saving. Asthma can be mild or severe, and at times can threaten life. In its worst expressions it can be seen to be a most frightening and exhausting experience. In acute stages it is folly to avoid the use of the life-saving potential of some of the medications available. Long-term use is, however, another story, and this is what the self-help methods would aim to replace.

Recalling the description of what occurs when a histamine reaction takes place, you can picture the constriction of the bronchioles, accompanied by a swelling of the local tissues. This is also accompanied by increased excretion of fluids by these tissues. This spasm, and additional obstruction caused by swelling and fluid excretion, results in great difficulty in breathing.

This is more marked in the exhalation phase of the breathing cycle. It is this that results in the characteristic wheezing and whistling type of breathing which asthmatics endure. The feeling that this engenders is one of suffocation. A degree of cyanosis may result from the retention of carbon dioxide and the consequent failure of adequate oxygenation. This gives a blue colour to the face of many asthmatics during an attack. Accompanying all this is the effort, on the part of the body, to expel the accumulating mucus excretions and, therefore, coughing attacks often accompany the gasping, breathing pattern.

The symptoms of asthma are only too familiar to many people. The acute distress is not easily forgotten.

As a general rule the onset of an attack is sudden, though premonitory symptoms (depressions, irritability and discomfort) may herald an approach. The asthmatic paroxysm usually asserts itself in the early hours of the morning. The patient awakens in an alarmed and anxious state, with a feeling of tightness and weight, and feels unable to expand his chest. The actual respiratory embarrassment may be preceded by sneezing or coughing. Acute discomfort is apparent, and respiration is only accomplished with difficulty, which produces the wheezing noises characteristic of asthma. The distress increases as the attack proceeds, and the patient tries to sit up with the shoulders raised and head thrown back, the whole body being torn with the desperate attempt to breathe. The pulse is rapid and weak and, while the extremities are cold, the face is wet with perspiration and either pale or livid. The patient's mind is set on breathing fresh air, and sufferers will often place themselves by an open window, irrespective of the cold. With the same desire for freedom and fresh air they loosen their clothing. The paroxysm lasts for a variable period - maybe for several hours. The easing of the attack is often marked by the expectoration of mucus and coughing. As the breathing becomes easier the sufferer recovers composure.

Frequent attacks of asthma are liable to produce emphysema, which is a condition where there is over-distension of the air-cells in the lungs, some destruction of tissue and the formation of large sacs.

These arise from the rupture, or combining together, of a number of adjoining air-vesicles. Bronchial asthma produces emphysema because, while obstruction prevents air from being expelled, inspiration is sufficiently forceful to overcome the obstruction, thus producing distension in the air cells. With persistent attacks of asthma the distension causes permanent change in structure, and emphysema results.

Asthma is often associated with bronchitis, nervous disease, and hay fever. Cardiac asthma consists of attacks of dyspnoea and cyanosis associated with palpitations and abnormally rapid action of the heart and pulse rate. Neither cardiac asthma nor renal asthma (difficult breathing in kidney disease) is a true asthmatic condition.

Broncho-dilators

The drugs used to treat asthma include what are known as broncho-dilators. These can be divided into two groups: those which are derived from theophylline and those from adrenaline. The adrenaline-like drugs are sympathomimetic; that is they have a stimulating effect which mimics that of the sympathetic nervous system. Among these substances are chemicals which are natural parts of the body's control mechanisms of the nervous system, adrenaline and noradrenalin (now also known as epinephrine and nor epinephrine).

These drugs attempt to alter the control of those parts of the body which are apparently out of control in the asthmatic attack. It would be too complicated to discuss all the many varied ways in which these drugs act, but here are some.

Depending upon which type of nerve ending is involved in treatment by a particular version of the sympathomimetic drug, the effect will vary. For example, those drugs which stimulate what are known as 'beta' receptors are used to treat obstruction to the airways, since they have a relaxing effect on bronchial muscles which are in spasm. Most drugs of this sort, however, also act on the heart, often causing serious coronary disorders, involving both the rate and rhythm of the heart. It has been noted that administration of such drugs (e.g. isoprenaline) by inhalant has actually increased the death rate from asthma amongst young people, as a result of this effect on the heart.

More selective forms of the drug are now available, such as Ventolin, which act on what are known as beta-2 receptors, and these have less harmful effects on the heart.

The other major group of drugs used in asthma are what are known as theophylline derivatives. These also act to produce relaxation of the bronchial muscles, and stimulate the centre in the brain responsible for breathing. A variety of side-effects have been associated with their use, including stomach irritation and vomiting. This is less likely if they are given by injection or suppository, but they may result in dizziness, nausea, rapid heart rate, and a fall in blood pressure, whatever method of administration is used.

In allergic asthma a drug called sodium cromoglycate (e.g. Intal) is used to interfere with the allergic reaction by stabilizing the mast cells and preventing release of histamine, but this is only effective if it is present in the lungs at the moment that the allergic reaction starts, and is of no use after it has begun.

The most dangerous of all medications used in asthmatic treatment are the hormonal drugs, the corticosteroids. These are used in severe acute attacks, when such injections can indeed save the life of the patient. Often in such situations they are used in combination with previously mentioned drugs. The dangers of long-term use of corticosteroids are many, and the use of them requires careful monitoring.

Fortunately medical science is now aware of the dangers, and there is a little chance of over-use or abuse of such drugs by reputable doctors.

Drug therapy for asthma deals with the symptoms, and not the causes, and can be most useful in crisis situations. Once established, a course of such drugs should be abandoned with utmost caution and under guidance from a qualified practitioner only. The idea is to avoid them if possible, and to provide the opportunity for a gradual weaning from them, by means of correction of the underlying causes, where this is possible. Even if it is not possible to totally reduce the use of drugs it should be possible to improve the state of health, and the condition itself, so as to allow for substantial reduction in dosage. The improvement that is possible in anyone case will differ from others, due to the many factors involved. The task we must face is to deal adequately with the various interconnecting aspects of the problem. We must begin to detoxify the system, improve nutritional status, reduce stress and tensions, improve environmental and atmospheric factors, improve overall function, and at the same time try to find safer alternatives for symptomatic relief. This is true of all allergic conditions, and not just the examples of hay fever and asthma which concern us at present.

My first consideration here will be to look carefully at detoxification and optimum nutrition.

4. Finding out to which foods you are allergic

The identification of foods to which we are sensitive can be difficult. In some cases it is obvious, and we therefore avoid the food. In other cases we may need to do long and difficult detective work in order to identify culprits. The self-help method that we will use first identifies those foods, or groups (families) of foods, which require further attention in our quest.

Make notes of the answers to the following questions

1. List any foods or drinks that you know disagree with you, or which produce allergic reactions (skin blotches, palpitations, feelings of exhaustion, agitation, or other symptoms).

2. List any food or beverage that you eat or drink at least once a day (or almost every day).

3. List any foods or drink that if you were unable to obtain, would make you feel really deprived.

4. List any food that you sometimes have a definite craving for.

5. If you are a nibbler between meals, what sort of food or drink is it that you use for such snacks? List these.

6. If there are any foods which you have begun to eat (or drink) more of recently, then list these as well.

7. Read the following list of foods and underline twice any that you eat at least every day, and underline once those that you eat fairly regularly, say three or more times a week:

Bread; milk; potato; tomato; fish; cane sugar or its products; breakfast food; sausages or preserved meat; cheese; coffee; rice; pork; peanuts; corn or its products; margarine; beetroot or beet sugar; tea; yogurt; soya products; beef; chicken; alcoholic drinks; cake; biscuits; oranges or other citrus fruits; eggs; chocolate; lamb; artificial sweeteners; soft drinks; pasta.

Pulse testing

Any food that is underlined should be added to your general list, derived from questions 1-6. If underlined twice, write it twice. Make a note especially of any food that appears on your list more than once as a result of the various questions. These are the most suspect foods, which we can try to identify by the following method, which is called 'pulse testing'.

What should you' do to discover the foods and substances to which you might be allergic? One of the simplest methods is to use Dr Coca's pulse test. Learn to take your pulse and keep a record of it for at least a week, testing it on waking, just before each meal, half an hour after each meal, and once more just before going to bed. If the pulse rate remains constantly below 84 per minute, then there is probably no allergy present. If there is a swing, up or down, of six or more beats per minute, then there probably is an allergy present. To test for suspected dietary allergens through the pulse test, miss a meal the night before, test the pulse on waking, then eat or drink a small quantity of the suspect food.

The pulse is then retested over the next hour or so. If there is any rapid rise of six or more beats per minute, or the onset of symptoms, then the test is positive. By working through all the suspect foods it should be possible to identify those which should be avoided, until the underlying problem has been corrected.

Unfortunately, there is sometimes a delayed reaction of 12 hours or more, and other factors can further confuse the picture, such as emotions, and the possible presence of hypoglycaemia (low blood sugar). The detective work might therefore prove difficult. Sometimes an arbitrary decision to eliminate a suspect item from the diet can be taken, just on the basis that it is easy to identify, and eliminate, for a test period of a few weeks.

One could therefore cut out all gluten-containing substances (wheat, oats, barley, rye) and see what happens to the symptoms. Similar elimination periods on a diet free of dairy produce, or fish, can be attempted. This method is hit and miss, but is often effective, especially when all dairy products are avoided. A range of gluten-free and dairy-free foods are now available from health stores. Eliminating from the diet those substances found to produce symptoms, or an increase in pulse rate, is certainly going to reduce symptoms and make for a more pleasant life.

Having eliminated the substances which cause a reaction, or a higher pulse rate, it is time to assess whether this has a marked effect on general health and/ or your symptoms. Of course, if it is not the hay fever season there may not be any symptoms anyway, but removal from the diet of the irritant food (the pulse rate would not rise if it were not an irritant) should help reduce the stress on the system, which would manifest itself in hay fever time as the onset of the symptoms.

There are other ways of reducing the stress of irritant foods, and one of these involves the use of a rotation diet, in which foods from any particular family of suspect foods are eaten only once in five days or so. This system is effective, especially if a detailed 'food and symptom diary' is kept, in which all deviations from your normal state of health are noted down as are all foods eaten. By comparing the two lists (foods and symptoms) it is often possible to note a pattern connecting particular foods and symptoms.

This really calls for the knowledge of a practitioner, and so it will not be detailed in this book. It could however aid the detective work that you have undertaken in this chapter if a diary were kept, as described above. Any obvious arrival of a symptom after a particular food could be noted, and that food removed from the diet.

Of course, the removal of such foods does little to correct the underlying sensitivity or allergic state. It is also obvious that many factors other than food can be responsible for allergic symptoms. We therefore should move onto a general detoxification programme, which will begin to tackle the needs of the body. In this detoxification programme any foods suggested which have appeared on the undesirable list, or which have provoked a rise in pulse rate, should be avoided.

After some months of detoxification, the pulse test can be tried again, and there may be a lessened or absent reaction, in which case a cautious reintroduction of the food can take place, perhaps no more frequently than once weekly at first.

I will now proceed to the task of detoxification and diet reform. It is true to say that much of the detective work described above would be unnecessary if the reforms suggested in the following chapter were introduced, because this would automatically cause the disappearance of the majority of refined, processed, stimulant, and junk foods. The substances which are found to give the most trouble to allergy victims are those which have been added to man's diet in the period of his adaptation from his early vegetarian mode of eating. These include flesh, fowl, dairy produce, cereals, modern processed foods, and all the added chemicals that these contain.

Detoxification and regeneration calls for a degree of discipline and effort. It is well worth the effort, for the result can be a greater sense of well-being and health than you ever dreamed possible.

Special note for asthmatics regarding sulphating agents

Substances known as sulphites are the commonest additive to food. They are added to most processed foodstuffs to delay their going off (thus prolonging their shelf-life). Foods, such as fruit juices, soft drinks, vinegar, potato chips, dried fruits, and fresh salad vegetables are often sulphated. The salads available at most salad-bars or restaurants may have had sulphite added, to keep them looking fresh. In the USA some states now demand that this information be clearly stated on menus. Many common medications contain sulphites and it is a common air pollutant. In the human lung there is an abundance of substances called prostaglandins, which convert inhaled sulphites from the atmosphere into a variety of substances which are toxic to the lungs. Asthmatics are known to be particularly susceptible to such irritation. Where possible, foods containing sulphites should be avoided. Careful reading of the labels on all processed foods should assist in this, as should care regarding use of medications containing these substances (most drugs used in die treatment of asthma paradoxically actually contain sulphites).

The overall detoxification programme described in the next chapter, together with the other methods outlined in the book, should reduce the level of sensitivity to this ubiquitous substance.

5. Detoxification and optimal nutrition for hay fever and asthma

In order to avoid recurrence of hay fever it is desirable to make a start well before the seasonal high point of pollen activity. It is not much use beginning a programme of detoxification and supplementation when the condition is already present. There are certainly a number of helpful things to be done at such a time, and these will be dealt with in Chapter 12. What we are looking at in this chapter are the long term dietary and nutritional methods which can help to prevent the next period of hay fever from happening, or at least to make it much less violent an experience, in people who are already victims of the condition. All the advice in this chapter is also applicable to asthmatics. The methods outlined below should therefore be started approximately six months prior to your usual hay fever season, whether this be a spring or autumn occurrence.

There are often variations in need, depending upon whether the irritant in your case is pollen or spores. Sensitivity to spores of fungi may indicate that there is an overall yeast intolerance, and we will look at some of the other symptoms which can confirm this, and an anti-yeast programme, at the end of this section. This is a possible involvement for both hay fever and asthma sufferers.

Asthma may be, and hay fever is always, an allergy, and as such we need to attempt to regenerate the immune function, and to detoxify, as much as possible, the organs and systems which are usually under some degree of toxic stress in such conditions.

The primary method of achieving this detoxification, and physiological regeneration, is by the use of either monodieting or fasting. This means spending a short period during which the body can eliminate accumulated materials which have built up due to a faulty dietary pattern, and poor eliminative function, often over a lengthy period of time. It is seldom desirable to undertake more than a few days at a time to this end, unless under a practitioner's guidance, and so a programme of repeated short fasts or monodiets (eating one food only for day or so) is called for. In therapeutic terms it is not a good idea to undertake a long fast without being under guidance or supervision of someone experienced in the methods. From a self-help point of view we can safely undertake a series of one or two day fasts (or monodiets) over a period of some months, with a fortnight or so in between. Thus it should be possible to arrange for a weekend twice a month, for a two or three month period, to be clear of social or other major obligations, during which time one of the methods outlined below can be put into operation.

Fasting

Fasting is the oldest therapeutic method known to man. Primitive people instinctively stop eating when not feeling well. In the same way, an animal that is ill will lie quietly, drinking as much as is needed, and eating nothing, until health returns. A fast is not starvation. The body has within it enough raw material to sustain life for many weeks, and in some cases for several months, without, any food at all. You may think that survival for months without food is unlikely; it is certainly unwise to contemplate, unless under expert supervision. Successful fasts, under controlled conditions, of over 100 days have been recorded.

However, a short fast of between two and four days is possible without supervision, if certain rules and advice are followed with care.

There is no cheaper, safer, or more effective way of achieving a revitalized, rejuvenated state of positive health than by fasting. There is also no more speedy and certain way of helping the body to cleanse itself of toxic wastes.

Fasting is the key to unlock many of the chronic problems that can hold our bodies in a vice of ill-health. Catarrh, chronic or acute, will respond with an increase in the elimination of catarrhal wastes, followed by an overall improvement. Digestive problems will respond to the physiological rest, with improved function. Rheumatic and arthritic conditions will respond with an increase in the elimination of acid wastes, followed by a lessening of pain and disability.

Almost all types of skin problems, from eczema to psoriasis to acne, will improve. The skin is one of the organs which show most dramatically the underlying state of the body. After a fast it is younger and more elastic, and has renewed tone. All allergic conditions improve with fasting.

Cautions

Do not fast without supervision if you have recently been, or are still taking drugs, in the treatment of any condition. Fasting is still desirable, even essential, in such a case, but not without the guidance of a naturopathic practitioner, or of a doctor who understands fasting.

• A diabetic should not fast without strict supervision.

• No-one who is highly-strung, or neurotic, should fast without guidance.

• Pregnant women should not fast, nor should a nursing mother, without expert advice.

• No-one should contemplate a long fast, say a week or more, unless they have experience of the method, or unless they are under' the care and advice of a practitioner.

The body repairs itself, given the chance. A cut will heal, a broken bone will knit and most 'acute' illnesses are self-limiting. The body can be seen to possess a built-in repair mechanism, which these examples illustrate.

This tendency to put things right, to normalize, to heal, is known as homoeostasis. Homoeostasis is constantly at work. Every activity of the body, and every change in its internal and external environment, causes the balancing mechanism to operate. If you walk out of a centrally heated room into the fresh night air, your body has to make rapid changes to cope with an alteration in external temperature. These changes involve the heart, circulation, muscles, etc., which will be 'tuned' to conserve body heat in the chilly exterior.

Go back into the hot room and everything goes into reverse; heat loss through the skin is now promoted, etc. All this is part of homoeostatic activity. You do not need to think about it, it just happens.

Many of the body's acute eruptions and eliminative efforts, such as colds, skin eruptions, diarrhoea, etc., are often no more than examples to the homoeostatic function of the body operating, in order to clear out toxic debris and waste material from the system. Any treatment which suppresses such acute episodes will only result in the body gradually becoming clogged with toxic wastes, and this will lead to chronic ill-health.

The day before the fast should be a raw food day, for example:

Breakfast: fresh fruit only (pear, apple, grapes, orange, etc.)

Mid-morning: fresh fruit or vegetable juice.

Lunch: Mixed vegetable salad (lettuce, cress, grated carrot, shredded cabbage, onion, pepper, grated raw beetroot, etc.) dressed with oil (e.g. sunflower) and lemon juice.

Mid-afternoon: fresh fruit or vegetable juice.

Evening: all-fruit meal.

The next day start fasting by following one of the methods described below.

Juice fast

On waking: hot lemon water (slice of lemon in tumbler, add hot water).

9 a.m. dilute apple juice or dilute orange juice, or dilute grape juice. (Juices should be homemade or additive free.)

11 a.m. dilute vegetable juice as above.

Alternate dilute fruit and vegetable juices every two hours, throughout the day. Dilution should be 50 per cent, with bottled spring water. Drink as much additional spring water as thirst dictates. If a hot drink is required have lemon water or herb tea (chamomile, peppermint, etc.) sweetened with a *very small* amount of honey. This can be maintained for two or three days, then the fast should be broken. You must be careful, as an unpleasant and sometimes dangerous reaction can follow if a 'normal' meal is eaten immediately after a fast.

The first meal should be either a bowl of fresh vegetable stew or soup (no condiments should be used in its preparation) or an apple or a pear, chewed thoroughly and slowly. A little natural goat's milk yogurt may be eaten at the same time as the fruit. The second meal can be the same, or a small mixed salad and a boiled or baked potato, all well chewed. Thereafter a return to a normal, food reform diet should be possible. This would include fruit and muesli for breakfast, a salad as one of the main meals and a protein (alternate days vegetarian, alternate. Days animal protein) and vegetable meal for the other main meal. All refined sugars and carbohydrates should be avoided, as should all tinned, processed or artificially flavoured foods. Tea, coffee, alcohol, etc. should be reduced to an absolute minimum.

Lemon and molasses fast

Recommended for anyone who is anaemic, or suffering from mineral deficiencies.

Every two hours during the day mix into a tumbler of warm spring water two tablespoons of molasses and two tablespoons of fresh lemon juice. Sip this slowly.

Maintain for two or three days. Break the fast as after, the juice fast. Drink spring water as thirst dictates,

Water fast

The simplest and quickest acting method is to remain on just water for the duration of the fast. Use spring water. Drink as much as thirst dictates, but not less than two pints during a 24-hour period.

What to expect on a fast

Hunger will not last for more than a day or so. The tongue will become heavily coated, and the urine dark and possibly foul smelling. This is evidence of elimination.

Clean your teeth regularly with a natural toothpaste to freshen the mouth. You will probably develop a headache which will clear after a day or so. Take nothing to stop this; it is dangerous to take drugs while fasting. You will need more sleep during a fast and should avoid excessive activity or stimulation. This does not mean that bed rest is necessary; by all means go for a walk and get some fresh air, but try to keep all activities low-key.

It is important to keep warm during a fast. Avoid draughts and put on an extra layer of clothing. A warm (not too hot) bath will assist in elimination through the skin, and will refresh you. Bathing morning and evening is quite in order.

Monodiets

Instead of a fast it is sometimes helpful to vary the pattern, and stay on just one food for a 24 to 48 hour period. Two of the most popular monodiets are the grape diet and the rice diet. In either case nothing else apart from the chosen food should be eaten, but as much spring water as desired can be consumed (not more than five pints a day though). On the days that one or other of these diets is to be followed, prepare the food in advance, so that as much rest as possible can be taken. The rice (whole brown rice) should be boiled and can be eaten hot or cold. It should be chewed extremely slowly, and *you* will find that a little goes a long way. Quantities depend on appetite, and the number of times it is eaten is also as variable as your desires. It is often found that having a few mouthfuls, six or seven times a day, is more desirable than trying to eat a meal of rice at set times. Allow your body to decide the pattern and quantity of the food eaten. With grapes the same applies. Eat little and often, or have a bunch at normal meal times, as desired. Eat slowly, chew well and try to eat the whole grape, seeds and all, if you can.

By either fasting or going on to a mono diet at least once, and ideally twice, a month, for 36 to 48 hours, a gradual lessening of the initial unpleasant symptoms will be noticed. This is a clear sign that detoxification is progressing, and that the fast is doing-its work. A different form of mono diet is to use a vegetable broth during the diet period. This is thin soup (see recipe in Chapter 5) which is consumed whenever hunger felt, in addition to whatever amount of water is drunk. The broth is light and nutritious and it can be eaten hot or cold, according to taste.

Use organically grown vegetables, if possible. If not, scrub the vegetables well before use. Into two quarts of spring water, place four capfuls of finely chopped beetroots, carrots, thick potato peelings, parsley, courgette and leaves of beetroot or parsnip. Use no sulphur-rich vegetables such as cabbage or onions, which might produce gas. Simmer for five minutes over a low flame, to allow the breakdown of vegetable fibre and the release of nutrients into the liquid. Cool and strain, using only the liquid and not the leftover vegetable content. Don't add salt, as this broth will contain ample natural minerals, providing nutrients without straining the digestive system. Also, it is alkaline and neutralizes any acidity resulting from the fast. Drink at least one pint of this nutritious broth daily during the fast. This broth can be used during a regular fast, or as a mono diet on its own.

In between the fast or mono diet periods the following general eating rules should be adopted, and the pattern of diet, as outlined below, should be followed as closely as possible. If anything on the dietary outline is known to be an irritant to you, or is something you do not enjoy eating, then adapt the pattern to your particular needs. In the previous sections we looked at some of the ways in which you might be able to identify for yourself foods to which you are sensitive.

Anything so identified should be dropped, as should the obviously undesirable factors discussed in point 6 below. This pattern of eating should be fully satisfying to you, and provides enough variations to allow for particular likes and dislikes. Six months of this diet should allow for a health regeneration after which modifications can be introduced.

1. Digestion begins in the mouth. Food should be eaten slowly and chewed thoroughly. .

2. Avoiding foods that are very hot or very cold will improve digestive functions.

3. Drinking any liquid with meals interferes with digestion, as does any liquid taken up to an hour after a main meal.

4. Simple meals without sauces are easier to digest.

Combinations of certain foods can produce indigestion, e.g. protein and carbohydrate do not mix well (bread and cheese, or fish arid chips).

5. Fried and roasted foods are difficult to digest, and should play only a small part in the diet.

6. Avoid completely:

• All white flour products, such as white bread, cakes, pasta, pastry, biscuits. Replace with wholemeal alternatives.

• All sugar of any colour, and its products, such as sweets, jams, soft drinks, ices, etc.

Replace with fruit, dried fruit, sugarless jam, fresh fruit juice, etc.

• Polished (white) rice. Replace with unpolished (brown) rice.

• Any foods containing additives, preservatives, colouring etc., such as most tinned foods.

• Tea, coffee, chocolate. Replace with herb teas, dandelion or other coffee substitutes.

• Strong condiments (vinegar, pickles, pepper, curry, etc.) Replace with herbs.

Reduce to a minimum the following:

• Alcohol (apart from a little wine).

• Milk, butter, cream and their derivatives. Use only low fat cheese, in moderation. Yogurt (if 'live') is acceptable, however.

• Margarine.

• Salt and salted foods.

• Meat. If animal protein is to be eaten then fish, chicken, eggs, etc. are more desirable than red meat, unless sensitivity is found to any of these.

7. The general pattern of eating should be as follows:

• Fifty per cent or more of the diet should comprise raw foods such as salad, fruit, seeds, nuts and cereals.

• Breakfast should be a fruit, seed, nut and cereal meal.

• One of the main meals should be a salad based meal with wholemeal bread, a jacket potato, or brown rice.

• The other main meal should contain a protein, either animal or vegetarian and vegetables.

• Desserts should be fresh or dried fruit. Snacks should be of fruit and seeds (sunflower etc.)

• Drinks should be between meals and be either fresh fruit or vegetable juice, spring water, a herb tea or coffee substitute, or a yeast type drink.

• One day each week should be a raw-food day (salads, fruit, seeds and nuts). This (or a fast or monodiet as described) should be extended to two days every six weeks or so, as a detoxifying period.

This type of diet, together with regular exercise, adequate rest and relaxation, and structural (mechanical) integrity, are the pre-requisites of health.

Digestive acids and asthma

It was noted in Chapter 2 that many of the problems relating to allergy in general, and asthma in particular, relate to imperfect digestion and absorption of foods, especially protein foods. When this happens it is often the case that partially digested particles enter the bloodstream and are reacted against by the body's defence mechanisms, triggering the symptoms of acute allergy. It has been observed for many years that this sort of imperfect digestion/ absorption can relate to an inadequate production by the body of hydrochloric acid, which plays a major part in the digestive process.

As far back as 1860 the following observation was made by a Dr Pridham, It appears to me probable that the original cause of the disease (asthma) was in the overworked powers of digestion.

Was it not probable that impurities in the blood were formed by imperfect digestion which were then thrown off by means of the lungs?

A Dr Salter noted in 1868, At times the precursory symptoms (of asthma) are connected with the stomach, and consist of loss of appetite, flatulence, costiveness and certain uneasy peculiar sensations in the epigastrium.

In 1931 Dr George Bray, writing in the quarterly *Journal of Medicine* stated, It has long been recognised that certain articles of diet disagree with certain asthmatics. Most sufferers evidence some manifestations of alimentary dysfunction such as vomiting, flatulence, 'liverish turns', constipation or bouts of mucous diarrhoea, and especially is this true of children.

We have already looked at methods of assessing which foods an asthmatic might be sensitive to, and the overall nutritional pattern which might be adopted in order to enhance health in general and digestive function in particular. In Chapter 7 we will examine certain nutrients which can assist in asthma and hay fever and one of these will be the use of hydrochloric acid, which has been noted to be on the low side in many asthmatics. This fact is put forward as a major element in the inadequate digestion of food, with the repercussions noted in Chapter 2.

Or Jonathan Wright makes an important observation in a 1986 article *(Health Consciousness,* Vol. 1 no. 4) when he declares,

In a study of 200 asthmatic children it was found that 80% were hypochlorhydric (low in hydrochloric acid), many severely. At my clinic we find this to be true with the highest percentage in the youngest age groups. It has long been known that hypochlorhydric patients do not absorb vitamin B12 as well as people with normal hydrochloric acid secretions.

This has led to the interesting research which has shown vitamin B12 to be a most useful substance in dealing with asthma, both acute and chronic. It also links with the use of pollen in such conditions (see Chapter 7) as asthma and hay fever, since this is rich in B12. Thus we have a picture emerging which points to weak digestive acids being the cause of inadequate breakdown of some foods, resulting in allergy as well as poor absorption of vitamin B12.

The poor digestive function is a key to the problem by increasing the chance of partially digested particles being absorbed, and this triggering an allergic response.

The B12 deficiency adds to the difficulty the body has in coping with this. It is clear therefore that part of a successful strategy should be to enhance digestive function. The dietary pattern suggested earlier will help in this direction, as will the supplements recommended in Chapter 7.

It is important in our dealing with the problem of asthma that overall dietary patterns be sound, with attention to removal of any obvious allergens from the diet. It is also obvious though that we need to deal with particular problems commonly found in people with this condition and inadequate digestive acid is one of those factors. Before moving on to look at supplementation we need to deal with another possible cause of digestive and other dysfunction, often noted in the problems of asthma and hay fever (and allergy generally) - this is the all too common infestation of the digestive tract by a parasite yeast, Candida albicans.

I have now outlined a general pattern of diet and detoxification, which can dramatically alter the tendency towards declining health. This gives the body a chance to begin to function normally again, and hopefully to reduce its sensitivity to irritant substances. We will now look at the possibility of yeast in general, and Candida albicans in particular, being factors in hay fever or asthma.

6. Is Candida an element in your condition?

Candida albicans is a yeast which inhabits parts of the body (usually the bowel, and sometimes the reproductive organs in women) *in every one of us.* Under certain conditions it has been shown to be able to spread well beyond these confines, especially if the immune function of the body is impaired. When this happens, it also has the chance to change into its fungal form (from its benign yeast state) and is capable of causing a wide variety of symptoms. Among these are certain allergic conditions. By answering the following series of questions you will be made aware as to the chances of this being the case in your condition. If spores are to blame for your immediate symptoms of allergy, whether asthma or hay fever, then the chance that you are 'yeast sensitive', is greater. If you are noticeably worse when in the proximity of a musty, mouldy environment, or when the weather is damp and muggy, or if the autumn is your worst time, this may well be the case.

There are no definite tests to prove Candida to be at fault in the system, because inevitably it is present in everyone. The degree of its involvement can be assumed by the number of positive answers given in the checklist below, and by adopting an anti-Candida programme it may be possible to prove this over a period of months, as the yeast activity, and therefore the symptoms, decrease. The dietary pattern suggested in the previous chapter is that indicated for Candida control, and the special supplements indicated (see below) will further aid this. The most specific variation in the diet for the Candida programme is total avoidance (if allergy is a problem), of all yeast based or fungus containing foods. A list of some of these will be found below.

Candida albicans checklist

The completion of this questionnaire will give clues as to whether Candida is an active agent in your current health spectrum. It is .not possible to make a diagnosis by these means alone, but a strong indication, as evidenced by positive answers in all sections of the questionnaire, is possible, and can be used to assist in deciding whether to undertake the Candida control programme.

History of drug usage etc.

1. Have you ever taken a course of antibiotics for an infectious condition which lasted for either eight weeks or longer, or for short periods four or more times in one year?

2. Have you ever taken a course of antibiotics for the treatment of acne for a month or more continuously?

3. Have you ever had a course of steroid treatment, such as prednisone, cortisone or ACTH?

4. Have you taken contraceptive medication for a year or more?

5. Have you ever been treated with immunosuppressant drugs?

6. Have you been pregnant more than once?

Major symptom history (Candida implicated)

1. Have you in the past had recurrent or persistent cystitis, vaginitis or prostatis?

2. Have you a history of endometriosis?

3. Have you had thrush (oral or vaginal) more than once?

4. Have you ever had athlete's foot, or a fungal infection of the nails or skin?

5. Are you severely affected by exposure to chemical fumes, perfumes, tobacco, smoke, etc?

6. Do you suffer from a variety of allergies?

7. Do you commonly suffer from abdominal distension, 'bloating', diarrhoea or constipation?

8. Do you suffer from premenstrual syndrome (fluid retention, irritability etc.)?

9. Do you suffer from depression, fatigue, lethargy, poor memory, or feeling of 'unreality'?

10. Do you crave for sweet foods, bread or alcohol?

11. Do you suffer from unaccountable muscle aches, or sensations of tingling, numbness, or burning?

12. Do you suffer from unaccountable aches and swelling in your joints?

13. Do you have vaginal discharge or irritation, or menstrual cramp or pain?

14. Do you have erratic vision or Spots before the eyes?

15. Do you suffer from impotence or lack of sexual desire?

If there are one or more positive answers to the first section and two 'or more in the second section, as well as some of the following symptoms being present then Candida is probably involved in your symptom causation.

Symptoms

Symptoms usually worse on damp days; persistent drowsiness; lack of co-ordination; headaches; mood swings; loss of balance; rashes; mucus in stools; belching and 'wind'; bad breath; dry mouth; postnasal drip; nasal itch and/ or congestion; nervous irritability; tightness in chest; dry mouth or throat; ear sensitivity.

If the indication is that you are a Candida subject then the diet should avoid (as well as those things discussed in the previous chapter) all foods containing, or based on, yeast. These include: all foods based on fermentation such as beer and wine; blue cheese; vinegar; dried fruit, mushrooms and anything extracted from yeast (such as Marmite).

Care should be taken' over the amount of bread and other 'yeasted' foods.

Supplements

The single most important supplement to aid the problem is the use of lactobacillus acidophilus. This is one of the friendly bacteria which inhabit the bowel.

Under normal conditions, it helps to control Candida but is rapidly destroyed by antibiotics. Among its many benefits to the body is its ability to produce one of the B vitamins, biotin. This is essential in the control of Candida; biotin slows down, or even prevents it from changing from the simple yeast form to the mycelial, invasive form. Acidophilus is sold in the US & UK in powder form, in extremely high dosages, as 'Superdophilus' and 'Vital Dophilus'. These products are often up to 800 times more powerful than standard acidophilus products. Vital Dophilus is suitable for anyone who is sensitive to dairy produce, which many

Candida sufferers are.

At the beginning of the treatment, up to a gram of one of these products should be taken daily for two weeks, followed by

500mg daily for at least six months. A 300-500mcg biotin tablet should be taken after each meal.

Garlic is also useful in controlling Candida. One excellent source, if you cannot bring yourself to eat a head of raw garlic each day, is the Japanese brand 'Kyolic'. One of the main ingredients of olive oil has a similar effect to biotin, and it is suggested that two dessert spoonfuls of cold pressed olive oil should be taken daily.

To help the immune system recover control over Candida, the amino acid arginine is recommended.

One or two grams should be taken daily on an empty stomach, unless you have a herpes problem, which would not respond well to arginine. Arginine is not recommended in these dosages if there is a history of schizophrenia, unless it is taken under supervision.

Other supplements that should be taken daily are one gram of vitamin C, a strong vitamin B-complex (from a yeast-free source) and 100mg of zinc orotate (B13 zinc).

In addition it has been noted that the juice of the desert plant Aloe Vera has strong anti-fungal effects, and a daily amount of two to three ounces of the juice of this plant should be consumed, if available (it is currently not on the UK market, but it is in the USA).

If Candida is a major problem, as indicated by the checklist, then a practitioner should be consulted regarding this.

7. Supplements to aid asthma and hay fever

The following food supplements can all aid the body, in one way or another, during the expression of an allergic reaction, and can also minimize the likelihood of a reaction occurring.

Hay fever

Pollen and hay fever protection

Pollen is an amazing complex of nutrients and has been shown to have protective effects against hay fever.

It contains all the water soluble vitamins, amongst them vitamin B12, of which more in Chapter 12. It also contains fat 'soluble vitamins such as E and K.

Minerals and trace elements are plentifully present as well as hormonal elements, which appear to be useful to humans. Interestingly, pollen contains all the essential amino acids necessary for human survival. If pollen from a good source is taken in tablet form for some weeks before the onset of the hay fever season, then it is found to minimize the intensity of the common symptoms, and often to prevent them altogether. Some of the finest sources of pollen derive from the Scandinavian countries, with the brand name 'Cernilton' being highly recommended. Health food stores should be able to supply these. Dosage of four to six pollen tablets daily are suggested, in a preventive role.

Vitamin supplements

The two most important supplements for use in dealing with hay fever are vitamin BS (pantothenic acid or calcium pantothenate) and vitamin C.

Vitamin BS is known to help the function of the adrenal glands, which are under stress in all allergic conditions. It is suggested that two 50mg tablets of this be taken daily, with food (as calcium pantothenate), during hay fever activity.

Vitamin C is a natural antihistamine and during the hay fever period it is suggested that no less than three tablets daily, of 500mg each, are taken with food. A higher dose is sometimes needed, and the tolerance level can be judged by the fact that when you are taking more than your body actually needs, diarrhoea will develop. If you gradually step up the dose to three or four grams a day, and no diarrhoea occurs, and your symptoms are under control, then maintain this during the sensitive period. When reducing dosage after the hay fever season, step the intake down gradually, by half a gram at a time for a few days, then again, until a maintenance dose of one gram a day is being taken.

The vitamin C taken should contain bioflavonoids.

This will be stated on the bottle.

The pantothenic acid can be taken at a dosage of 50mg daily during the period of the diet as outlined previously, and at 100mg daily when hay fever is current.

These supplements have specific effects on the physiology of the body, and are part of the overall programme, rather than 'cures' in their own right. It is important to tackle underlying causes, via detoxification and stress reduction etc., and not just to rely on 'remedies'.

It has been noted in many hay fever cases that the individual (especially in children) is deficient in hydrochloric acid secretions. This factor and notes on supplementation, is discussed below.

Asthma

As noted in Chapter 5, there is a strong connection between deficiency of hydrochloric acid and mal-absorption problems, which can lead to both deficiency of vitamin B12 and allergic responses to partially broken down proteins, which are absorbed into the bloodstream via the digestive tract. Studies have shown that in any group of asthmatic children, around 10 per cent are very low in hydrochloric acid production (in some none being found at all, after meals); around 50 per cent show marked reduction in normal levels of hydrochloric acid; and over 20 per cent show a mild degree of hypochlorhydria. This means that around 80 per cent of asthmatic children will be found to need supplementation with hydrochloric acid tablets.

Age seems to be a factor, in that the younger the patient the more marked the deficiency. Few studies have included many adults - those which do show mixed results, with some individuals showing marked improvements and others none in response to added hydrochloric acid. As children grow so does their level of acid, increase. This correlates with the often observed factor of 'growing out of the allergy. In many instances the more severe cases of deficiency of hydrochloric acid noted in children commenced soon after a serious episode of a childhood disease, such as measles, which resulted in bronchopneumonia. Similar tests on hay fever sufferers indicates low hydrochloric acid levels, although the degree of deficiency does not seem as dramatic as in asthma sufferers. When a group of normal (i.e. no allergy) children are examined in this manner only about 10 per cent of these show low levels of hydrochloric acid.

Supplementation of hydrochloric acid is by tablet. It is most important that these are swallowed and not chewed, as the acid will damage the teeth if it comes into direct contact with them. As a rule tablets are prepared in doses of around 300mg (Betaine Hydrochloride) and are often combined with the substance pepsin (in a dosage of around 5mg), another of the secretions of the stomach involved specifically in protein digestion. Between one and three such tablets are taken at each meal, with food, but not chewed.

It has been found that if hydrochloric acid supplementation is introduced together with removal of substances to which allergy has been shown (see Chapter 4) then results are very speedy in reducing intensity and frequency of asthma attacks. If this is begun early in the season during which asthma is at its worst (usually, but not always, winter) and continued for some months, until a period of several months without attacks has passed, the use of HCl may then be discontinued. Often this leads to a situation in which attacks cease altogether. This is more likely if the overall strategy of dietary intake, as outlined previously, is adhered to, and those foods which have shown to be allergens are avoided, or kept to a minimum. There is usually a noticeable increase in appetite and energy, and improvement in sleep patterns, when this programme is begun.

When only hydrochloric acid is used, and no attention is paid to dietary exclusion of allergens, the improvement noted is less, although still marked.

Attacks tend to continue, but at reduced rate and intensity. This approach, however, is not one which can be left off without risking a return to severe asthma attacks, and so is not recommended. Both supplementation and dietary control are required for good permanent results. Reports indicate that the use of hydrochloric acid supplementation in hay fever sufferers produces very good results indeed, with over 70 per cent of patients in one study having complete remission from symptoms during the hay fever season.

Betaine Hydrochloride with Pepsin is available from a good health food store.

Other nutrients and asthma

Vitamin B6, or pyridoxine, is involved in the synthesis in the body of many important neurotransmitter substances. In asthmatics it has been demonstrated that levels of B6 are significantly lower than in normal individuals, and the taking by mouth of 50mg daily of this vitamin has been sufficient to dramatically diminish the frequency of asthma attacks, and also to reduce the severity of wheezing. Thus the role of taking of this vitamin is not as a treatment of the symptoms, although these are helped, but rather as a making good of a deficiency of a substance, which has some bearing on the underlying condition.

This distinction is important since we must know whether we are trying to deal with causes or with symptoms. There is no harm whatever in using safe measures to reduce the intensity of symptoms, especially when they are so ghastly as in asthma.

However such short-term measures, some of which are described in Chapter 12, will never normalize the problem, whereas dealing with causes may.

Vitamin C and asthma

Vitamin C has also been demonstrated as being in short supply in asthmatics, both treated and untreated.

These deficiencies were found in the bloodstream and in cells. It has been found that when' artificial means are used to constrict bronchial tissues, vitamin C prevents this in normal individuals as well as in asthmatics. A variety of tests have demonstrated that sometimes small amounts of additional vitamin C can act to prevent asthmatic symptoms in certain people, whereas in others a large amount is required to achieve the same result. This relates to what is known as biochemical individuality.

This concept was proved by Professor Roger Williams of Texas University. He showed that in any group of people in perfect health, there is a demonstrable variation of up to 500 per cent in the individual needs for certain vitamins, minerals, etc. Thus one person may require up to five times as much vitamin A as another, and someone else might need three or four times the calcium and/ or magnesium as do others.

This individualized need for any nutrient is seen to be genetically controlled, and to be a major reason for variations in the way we respond to diets and supplementation.

It requires, therefore, that we should attempt to discover, by trial and error very often, what our needs really are in nutrient terms. As far as vitamin

C is concerned there are methods of establishing accurately whether the body has enough to meet its needs. One such method is the use of a tongue test in. which a drop of a harmless liquid is placed on the centre of the tongue, and the time it takes to disappear (it is purple) is measured. If this is 15 seconds or less

there is adequate vitamin C in the body; if over 20 seconds then there is inadequate vitamin C present. By taking some supplemental and testing again, the correct level can be established.

Another method is that mentioned briefly earlier in this chapter (under the heading Hay fever). This is the process developed in California by Or Robert Cathcart, in which there is a step-by-step increase in the amount of vitamin C taken in supplement form by a gram a day at a time until a level is reached which provokes mild diarrhoea. This indicates bowel tolerance has been reached, and that the amount being taken is too much. By reducing to the previous day's intake level, the amount required currently by the body is established, as evidenced by normal bowel function returning.

There can be many reasons for variations in requirement for vitamin C (and other nutrients) other than inborn tendencies. Stress, for example, puts up the need for C greatly, as does exposure to pollution, infection, allergy, and pregnancy. By establishing the true needs of the body, by testing bowel tolerance in this manner, or by tongue testing, and by meeting these needs, the body will be better able to cope with its defensive functions. Protection against the worst of asthmatic (and hay fever) symptoms is noted when approximately one gram daily (on average since, as explained, requirements will vary) is taken.

Antioxidants and asthma

A number of nutrients such as vitamins A and E and the mineral selenium are known as antioxidants (vitamin

C is also one of these). This indicates that they have the ability to prevent or reduce the processes of oxidation which take place in the body as a result of the presence of irritant substances. When an apple is peeled and exposed to the air it oxidizes and turns brown. If lemon juice (rich in vitamin C) is squeezed over it this slows down the oxidation process. Similarly in the body a number of continuous processes occur in which certain substances oxidize. As they do so, some can produce what are called free radicals, and these can be extremely damaging and irritating to healthy tissues. It is the group of nutrients mentioned (and others) which act to protect the body. In allergic reactions this process is heightened and the need for additional protective nutrients is greater. Thus an intake of vitamin A in the form of carotenes (the substances which the body turns into vitamin A) as well as vitamin E and selenium, are recommended in doses of:

Carotenes up to 100,000 iu (international units) daily Vitamin E 400 iu daily Selenium 250 micrograms daily.

Magnesium and asthma

As long ago as 1912, scientists demonstrated that the mineral magnesium relaxed bronchial smooth muscles. These are the muscles which contract and make breathing so difficult in asthma. The benefits of using magnesium were later demonstrated in patients with bronchial asthma, and were it not for the arrival on the scene of hormone drugs such as cortisone, and other powerful medications (often with side-effects), the use of magnesium in asthma might now be standard procedure. Unfortunately this safe line of research was dropped. However, with the arrival of even newer drugs called calcium channel blockers for the treatment of asthma, renewed interest has been stirred in magnesium, which is a natural antagonist of calcium activity. Trials in 1985 indicated that use of magnesium (in injection form) significantly improved the function of breathing in asthmatics. There is no reason why the taking of magnesium by mouth should not also be beneficial, although it will not act as rapidly as the injected forms. A daily dosage of 500mg of magnesium is suggested for asthmatic individuals during periods of likely attack.

8. Stress reduction for asthma and hay fever

The environment in which relaxation exercises are practised should be quiet and not unduly warm or cold. The surface on which the exercise is performed should be firm, but not so hard as to be uncomfortable or so soft as to induce sleep. A blanket on a carpeted floor is perhaps the ideal surface. Clothing should be loose, with no constricting or distracting elements.

Remove shoes, ties, etc. and undo bras and belts.

Lying on the back is the ideal position, with a small neck pillow, and a bolster or cushion under the knees if the back is more comfortable that way. (Anyone who has a history of low-back strain, or who has a hollow back, will probably be more comfortable with the knees slightly flexed, in this way). Sitting in a supported position is suggested if there is any tendency to fall asleep when in the lying position.

Some adepts at yoga prefer the cross-legged or lotus position, and others prefer to kneel, using a small stool to support the buttocks. Whichever position is chosen, the only essential aspect, as far as the first two exercises are concerned, is that you are comfortable. Later exercises will specify if a particular position is desirable. Falling asleep during the performance of any exercise is to be avoided since the aim is to practise and experience something consciously.

There should be no distracting sounds, such as radio or T.V., during the relaxation period, and no sense of urgency should be felt. It is probably best not to attempt such exercises too soon after eating a meal.

Morning and evening seem to be times that suit most people. Once you have introduced your routine, endeavour not to miss practising the exercises, for it is only by persistent repetition that the first stages of relaxation will be mastered, leading on to deep relaxation and other methods of 'mind control'. At first it may appear that nothing much is happening. Indeed the tense individual probably believes deep down that such simple measures, helpful as they may be to others, are not for him with his super active mind which just cannot relax. Patient, persistent and thorough application will satisfy even this type of individual that the methods are worthwhile.

When you begin to practise any relaxation exercise, you will find that intrusive thoughts come periodically into the mind to interrupt the smooth flow of the technique. This is normal and to be expected. It should not produce any reaction of distress or anger. When a thought intrudes, push it gently to one side and resume the exercise. It does not matter how frequently such interruptions occur, simply carry on where you left off.

Gradually, week by week, there will be fewer interruptions and relaxation will deepen. Whichever exercise is being used, there should be an awareness that there is no 'correct' response. Your body and your mind will respond *your* way. Be passive and do not 'force' the exercise. Relaxation comes at its own speed. Be an observer of the processes taking place; sense changes which occur in a detached way. Let things happen and register your thoughts and feelings. Above all be patient and passive.

Rhythmic abdominal breathing

Whilst learning the technique, arrange to have two free periods per day, each of five to fifteen minutes. Find a quiet room where you know you will not be disturbed.

Rest on your back, head and shoulders slightly raised, pillow under the knees to take the strain off them and off your back. Rest your hands on the upper abdomen, close your eyes, and settle down in a comfortable position.

See that there is nothing in the room that is going to distract your attention, such as sunlight, a clock, animals, and so on. Sitting in a reclining position is also suitable, and many people prefer this to lying down. Try both and choose whichever is most comfortable.

Attention to breathing is of great value in relaxation, particularly during the initial stages. The person who is at ease with himself and the world breathes slowly, deeply, and rhythmically. Breathing is the only automatic function which one is capable of controlling. It is carried out partly through the autonomic nervous system and partly through the central nervous system.

The autonomic nervous system is that which controls vital functions, endocrine (hormone) secretions and emotions. By controlling one's breathing, one can influence all these and for a short time take over conscious responsibility for them.

The aim is to breathe slowly, deeply and rhythmically.

You cannot expect to do this perfectly to begin with - it might even take weeks. Inhale through the nose slowly and deeply. The abdomen, on which the hands are resting, should rise gently as the breathing begins. An awareness of this rising and falling of the abdomen is important to establish that the diaphragm is being used properly. The inhalation should be slow, unforced and unhurried. Whilst breathing in, silently and slowly count to four or five. When the inhalation is complete, pause for one or two seconds, then slowly exhale through the nose. As you exhale, you should feel the abdomen slowly descend. Count this breathing out, as you did when breathing in.

(Again, a count of four or five should be achieved.)

The exhalation should take at least as long as the inhalation.

There should be no sense of strain regarding the breathing cycle. If, at first, you feel you have breathed to your fullest capacity by a count of three, then so be it. Try to gradually slow down the rhythm until a slow count of five (or even six) is possible, both on inhalation and exhalation, with a pause of one or two seconds between. Remember to start each breath with an upward push of the abdomen. With the mind thus occupied on the mechanics of the breathing, as described above, as well as on the rhythmic counting, there is little scope of thinking about anything else.

Nevertheless, initially at least, extraneous thoughts will intrude. This pattern of breathing should be repeated 15 to 20 times and, since each cycle should take fifteen seconds, this exercise should occupy a total of about five minutes.

It is suggested that during the exercise, once the mechanics and counting have become well established as a pattern, it is useful to introduce a variety of thoughts during different phases of the cycle. For example, on inhalation try to sense a feeling of warmth and energy entering the body with the air. On exhaling, sense a feeling of sinking and settling deeper into the supporting surface. An overall sense of warmth and heaviness, accompanying the repetitive breathing cycle, will effectively begin the relaxation process.

Physiologically ~ this exercise will slow down the heart rate, reducing sympathetic nervous activity ~ relax tense muscles, and allow a chance for the balancing, restorative parasympathetic nervous. Function to operate, as well as calming the mind. In the initial stages this is sufficient exercise for one session.

When proficient, it can be used to precede other relaxation methods and, later in a shortened version of, say eight to ten breathing cycles, a meditation or visualization technique.

After completion of the exercise, do not get up immediately but rest for a minute or two, allowing the mind to become aware of any sensations of stillness, warmth, heaviness, etc. Once mastered, this exercise can be used in any tense situation with the certainty that it will defuse the normal agitated response and should result in a far greater ability to cope.

The relaxation method described above is ideal for an asthmatic when not in the midst of an attack. Once mastered, the abdominal breathing pattern can be used during an attack to facilitate the breathing which is laboured. Hay fever victims should employ the same methods.

Stress reduction

Overall stress reduction demands attention to lifestyle.

You should include adopting a pattern of life which incorporates the following:

• Avoid working more than ten hours daily and ensure that you have at least 1 1/2 days a week free from routine work. If at all possible, an annual holiday 'away from it all', should be arranged.

• During each day, have at least two relaxation or meditation periods. Time should be set aside morning and evening, or just prior to a meal.

• Perform active physical exercise for at least 10 minutes daily, or for 20 minute periods, four times each week.

• Balance the diet and eliminate stress-inducing foods and drinks.

• Try to move, talk, and behave in a relaxed manner.

• Seek advice about any sexual or emotional problems that are nagging away at the back of your, mind, or which are causing conscious anxiety.

• If there are actual stress-inducing factors at work or home which can be altered, then make concrete steps towards these changes.

• Cultivate a creative rather than a competitive hobby, e.g. painting, DIY, gardening, etc.

• Try to live in the present, avoiding undue reflection on past events or anticipating possible future ones.

• Concentrate on whatever the current task is, always finishing one thing before starting another.

• Avoid making deadlines or 'impossible' promises that could lead to stress. Take on only what you can happily cope with.

• Learn to express feelings openly in a non-belligerent way, and in turn, learn to listen carefully to other people.

• Accept personal responsibility for your life and health - don't look outside yourself for causes or cures, apart from the objective guidance and practical advice available from a health professional.

• Greet, smile and respond towards people in the same way that you would like to be treated.

• Introduce negative ionization into the home or work place and ensure adequate exposure to full spectrum light.

Take several months to introduce all these changes.

9. Guided imagery and self healing

After learning the breathing (relaxation) exercise, and practising it for several weeks, introduce the methods described below, in which guided imagery (or visualization) is used to help you to overcome whatever physical ailment is manifesting itself, be it asthma, hay fever, or anything else.

The term 'psychosomatic' is now one in common use, and the idea that the body can indeed become sick as a result of the negative influence of the mind is no longer in any doubt. There is plenty of evidence that many diseases, both acute and chronic, mild and serious, have at their root psychosomatic, or mind induced, causes.

So, if this is generally accepted, then surely it is but a short step to accept the converse: that the mind is capable of exerting beneficial effects as well as harmful ones. There is constant research and debate about just how much influence the mind has over the body, and the probability is that it varies depending on personality, behaviour and beliefs. So the same stresses in two different people will not produce the same health problems. It is also true that identical symptoms, asthma for instance, may have quite different origins.

The potency of the mind to heal should not be underestimated. It is all a matter of reversing its negative, destructive ability, and the key to this lies in learning to replace harmful patterns of thought and images with positive, helpful, and healing ones. This in fact is the basis of guided imagery or visualization. For this it is essential, first of all, that the individual is in a state of deep relaxation. Then, by using one of the various methods of meditation, the mind can be taught to focus on a single object, idea or thought, to the exclusion of all others.

The potency of this technique is vouched for by its large scale use in the treatment of cancer, for example.

Through positive imagery, as well as other therapeutic measures, cancer, and other chronic degenerative diseases, have frequently been controlled and 'cured'.

The key to this success lies in the images that the mind is asked to project, and in the state of relaxation achieved prior to this being done. The other major element is regular repetition of the exercise. It is no use doing it sometimes, or just when symptoms are at their worst. It is necessary to perform the exercise regularly and to be in a state of relaxation when doing so. It is also essential to have an image of the part of the body which needs to be influenced by this exercise.

One of the major elements in visualization is learning to relax. The method is unimportant, as different approaches suit different people. Meditation teaches the mind to focus upon one object or thought without distraction. The benefits of meditation are well documented, and include the reduction of excessive nervous activity, the lowering of blood pressure, and the general balancing of the physiological state of the body.

Transcendental meditation

While the best known methods of meditation are those taught by the Maharishi and his followers (transcendental meditation or TM), it is now well established that these are not the only ones which can achieve successes. Basically, TM teaches a system in which individuals begin by using a repetitive sound, which they silently repeat to themselves as they progressively relax and still their minds from its normal chatter. The sound (or mantra) is given to the trainee meditator, and is said to be selected specifically to meet his/her particular personality and needs. It is a meaningless (to the western mind) sound, 'Om', 'Ram', etc., which, on repetition, becomes a sort of thought-blanketing drone in the mind, and which helps to still all other thoughts.

By regularly practising this method the meditator can achieve dramatic health improvements, as well as finding a greater ability to concentrate, new energy levels, improved sleep patterns, and so on. The need of secret mantras is questioned by many, however. They say any sound or idea (love, God, etc.) or image (circle, candle flame, cross, etc.) or phrase ('God is love' etc.) will suffice. Indeed, it has been seriously suggested that the use of words such as 'Coca-Cola' or 'bananas', repeated silently as the individual sits or lies in an undistracting environment, will do just as well as anything else.

Guided visualization

If good use is to be made of the amazing power of the mind then it should be harnessed and directed towards positive health achievements, and whether the problem is one of an illness (circulatory problems, ulcers, bronchial disease, arthritis, etc.) or a desire to break bad habits (such as smoking, overeating, alcohol) or just to improve well-being (to become more confident, more relaxed and loving, etc.) then these methods of meditation and relaxation should be used. There is no doubt the mind can heal, and we must use this ability.

'All it takes is a little learning and application. It costs nothing but our own effort, and the rewards are immeasurable. Relax in a quiet room using a method (such as that described in the previous chapter) that most suits you, in order to induce a sense of ease.

Spend two or three minutes in safe, peaceful and harmonious contemplation. You are now ready for guided visualization to promote healing.

Create in your mind a picture of any illness or ailment you have. This should be done in a way that makes sense to you. It does not have to be scientifically accurate. Examples are given below of how this might be done. Having visualized your ailment, illness, or condition, try to see your body's defence and healing mechanisms overcoming, controlling or correcting the condition.

See, for example, the lungs and the network of tubes, being irritated by mucus deposits. See the mucus being cleared away by the body, and see the air passages cleared and, expanding to allow a free passage of air. Visualize the removed debris being easily coughed up, and then picture the soft mucous membrane lining the air passages as producing just enough clear liquid to lubricate the movement of surfaces. See the lungs expanding and contracting to their full capacity. See yourself walking, running, or enjoying any activity that is difficult at present.

Keep it firmly in your mind that there are few, if any, conditions which cannot be improved, controlled or normalized by the self-healing mechanisms of the body. If any treatment is being undertaken to help the condition, visualize this too, in whatever way makes sense to you. *Know* that you will be well again. See yourself well, healthy, free of pain or discomfort; visualize yourself being active and doing something pleasant, such as walking in a meadow, or swimming in the sea. Imagine yourself achieving something you have as a goal in life. Feel satisfied and content that you are, in this way, able to support and participate consciously in your recovery.

When you have completed the visualization, either rest for a while or resume your normal activities. Do this exercise two or three times daily, as well as, or instead of, your relaxation programme. Two to ten minutes of this imagery should be performed on each occasion.

Any ailment or condition can be approached this way, and negative thoughts, doubts, and fears can thus be overcome. A sense of being in control of the healing process brings with it self-confidence and hope; the will to live, and determination not to give in, the knowledge that you are working with your body, and with the healing process - all these factors are enhanced, and are of immeasurable value. Physical changes can stem directly from guided imagery of this type. Believing in one's recovery makes it all the more likely and speeds up the process.

It is not possible for everyone to visualize pictures of the sort described. In some cases, people just cannot think in this way, and in such cases, picturing words or feelings is perfectly adequate.- Remember that the exercise is flexible enough to be used by anyone. It is a matter of seeing the problems your way, and imagining the way in which the body, sustained by treatment, may overcome it. All these should be in images, words, or feeling that makes sense to you.

• The illness must be seen as a weak vulnerable enemy.

• The body's defence capacity must be seen as strong and easily capable of destroying and removing the enemy deposits in arteries, tumour cells, mucous congestion, etc.

• Previously damaged areas must be thought of as easily repaired by the body, and should be seen as normal again. Oversensitive tissues are seen as normal again.

• Any debris from the healing process is thought of as easily cleared from the body and should be seen as flushed away.

• Any treatment should be seen as supporting the powerful healing mechanisms, and providing an even more certain end to the problem.

When doing the visualization exercise the words used to affirm 'wellness' can be adapted to you particular beliefs. A number of medical practitioners now use the words first described by the American healer Louise Hay, in which she related particular affirmations to particular conditions. The affirmation for asthma is 'I am free. I take charge of my own life'. Much psychological work in asthma has related the condition, in many cases, to a feeling of being smothered or stifled by life's events or situations, and often to represent a suppressed crying. The relaxation and visualization, accompanied by the positive affirmation of freedom, will aid in overcoming such deep seated emotional feelings if they are present.

In hay fever the affirmation, which can be part of the visualization or which can simply be mentally repeated whenever a moment permits, is, 'I deny all beliefs in calendars. I am one with ALL life'. This is obviously meant to instil a feeling of being impervious to the seasonal cycles of the condition. If preferred, the affirmation for allergy can replace either of those already mentioned. This is 'I am at peace. The world is safe and friendly'. Hay fever is seen as representing 'emotional congestion', and allergy a false ego and sensitivity.

The overall importance of lifestyle reform, and the taking of regular physical exercise, such as walking, cannot be overemphasized. The regular performance of the breathing-relaxation exercise, and the subsequent visualization, is highly recommended. There are other forms of relaxation which suit individual needs better than the methods described above, but these are by far the easiest to learn and to apply, without personal instruction.

In Chapter 11 we will consider a method of atmospheric or environmental adjustment, which is of paramount importance, especially in polluted city environments.

This is the use of ionizers. Before that, however, we will take a brief look at the needs of the asthmatic or allergic child.

10. The asthmatic child

We have tended to pay great attention thus far to the physical needs of the asthmatic individual, and this is a valid approach since it oft-times achieves relief and removal of the symptoms of asthma. The relaxation and meditation methods, as outlined in the previous chapter, are useful for all individuals with asthma, although it is not easy to teach children all the finer points of these methods. Just how important mental ease is in asthma has been demonstrated in a number of well conducted research studies involving asthmatic children. One *Journal of Psychosomatic Research,* vol 29, no 2, pp 177-182} found an extraordinary link between parentally induced stress and asthma, so that when children with asthma were removed from their parents for a while (only half jokingly called 'parentectomy') the symptoms decreased dramatically. The factors involved were ascertained by use of careful interviews and questionnaires.

This helped to identify many personality characteristics in the parents of nearly 200 children with asthma, including many examples of 'aggression', guilt feelings, dominance, etc. The characteristics which predominated were that parents of asthmatics tended to be more aggressive, and less open in their demonstrations of feelings. The definition of 'aggressive' in this context meant that these were commonly people who sought to take 'revenge' when insulted; to take pleasure in irritating people they disliked; to want to break things and to lose their tempers easily; and to find other people irritating. They tended not to want to be the centre of attention and to be retiring, unless provoked.

Parents of asthmatics were often dominated by these characteristics, and it was often the case that the mother was the main organizer of the two parents, taking decisions etc. There was a common thread amongst many parents of having initially rejected the child, for one reason or another, which was followed by feelings of guilt and an overcompensation which led to overprotection. .The combination of overprotection, combined with a degree of rigidity in displaying feelings, and a tendency to rage when provoked, were all unhelpful to the child. When an asthmatic child from such a background was taken on holiday, or to stay with other relatives for a while, the symptoms of asthma declined dramatically, despite all other factors staying the same. Thus diet was unchanged, exposure to irritant fumes of pollution was unchanged, physical factors were the same, etc., but mental stresses were different and the symptoms responded by going away.

This must give cause to any parent to consider whether they are being overprotective, lacking in displays of inner feeling, and/or liable to fly off the handle too easily. It is also clear from this that there are many parents in whom these characteristics do not apply. They were, however, found to apply more strongly and more often, than in parents of normal children.

In trials which looked at the way asthmatic children themselves reacted to events it was found that, in comparison to normal children, they had a strong tendency to retain their emotions, not showing what they felt. Specifically the frequency and duration of expressed anger/rage, or enjoyment/joy, or even of being startled or surprised, were very much less obvious, under appropriate conditions, in asthmatic children. This could of course have been a learned response ~in that having parents who did not show joy, anger, surprise, etc. had led to their doing the same thing. It was considered by the researchers (in Germany) that there was a strong degree of correlation between the lack of facial expression in such children, and the degree of rigidity in their breathing function.

What is to be done about such factors? It is difficult for individuals and families to first of all recognize that their own unconscious behaviour could be the cause of distress and illness in loved ones. This is the first hurdle to be crossed, since no progress can be made without recognition of the factors involved. It must initially be made absolutely clear that no attempt is being made to 'blame' people for such attitudes and behaviour patterns.

These are the result of learned responses, and in order to change them they need to be looked at and changed by consciously understanding how and why they exist. Why is this person or that person unable to easily demonstrate their emotions? Why is anger so quick to surface? Why is there so little facial expression?

How does change come about? It is of course not suggested that self-treatment is possible or even desirable in such a complex area. Awareness of the research findings mentioned can, however a trigger a change in itself, but it is probable that counselling, guidance and even psychotherapeutic advice is needed to overcome deep-seated ways of dealing with life. That it is desirable and necessary for change to be made is obvious from the nature of the problem being discussed.

Asthma is horrible, and efforts to overcome it require looking at all avenues. It should be obvious from this discussion that any attempt to improve nutritional status, or to make any other desirable changes, in a child, should be accomplished with a great deal of care, and not by introducing factors which will increase stress and anxiety. Perhaps the best approach in children is to explain fully the reasons why changes are being made; and to avoid dogmatic and harsh attitudes as to what is eaten, etc. Explanation and care, in a loving environment, will go a long way to helping the situation, as will reduction of overall stress via the methods discussed in the previous section.

The child with asthma or hay fever

Much of the advice and instruction given in the chapters on diet depend upon an understanding of the association between nutritional factors and the allergic state. The specific possibility of food allergy being part of hay fever or asthma exists, and this requires an understanding and responsible attitude towards eating correctly. For a child, especially a young one, there is little chance of such awareness, and the parental role is made doubly difficult by the effort required in attempting to control childhood wants and desires.

This can be stressful to parent and child, and of course stress is not desirable in the circumstances of acute allergy, especially asthma. There is unfortunately no easy answer, and my advice to parents is to stick as closely as possible to the guidance given regarding food without making life intolerable for all concerned.

One way of depriving a child of desired, yet undesirable, food is just not to have it in the house. Sugary, sweet foods and pastries, cakes, tinned and 'chemicalized' foods can be avoided by the simple expedient of not buying them. Fried foods can be avoided by not cooking that way, and the use of dairy produce cut down by careful menu adjustments. There are desirable alternatives for almost all the junk foods that children want, and sensible searching through available whole food cookbooks will yield many wholesome surprises.

This is the task for the caring parent, and it should be accomplished with a minimum of fuss and bother, so that if a favourite food simply 'disappears', it is replaced by something else which is desirable and nutritious. As mentioned, it is not a particularly easy task, though not impossible.

For the allergic child, though, the inhaled substance is often as harmful as the eaten substance. In the case of hay fever and asthma this aspect requires a common-sense approach, and the following general instructions should contain some advice which is pertinent to your particular needs. Anything that encourages dust retention in the home, and especially in the child's room, should be removed. This includes rugs and curtains (blinds may be better). Ensure that mattresses, bedding, and pillows contain no feathers, and that the room is kept as dust-free as possible. It is possible to obtain dust-proofing material to cover beds, mattresses, and pillows, and also dust-proofing liquid with which to cover the surfaces in a child's room. This helps to prevent dust from accumulating.

These products are available in the USA.

Children with asthma should be kept away from dusty and musty places, such as attics and cellars. Soft toys are also a potential hazard, as they may be stuffed with undesirable materials. Pillows, etc. should be made from dacron, or an odourless rubber material.

Any chemical fumes are a danger to the allergic child, and so petrol, cleaning fluids, paint, and all household chemicals and sprays, as well as plastic glues, should be avoided in the home as much as possible.

Animals may present a further complication, and the sensitive child should not play with pets, be they birds or four legged animals. Such pets should be kept out of the child's room, and if definite reaction to animals is noted, then no pets should be kept in the home.

Many common drugs trigger allergies, and so aspirin and antibiotics especially should not be used without a doctor's instruction.

If pollen is the key to the child's problem the avoiding of gardens and countryside, especially during the spring, is an obvious measure. In all hay fever and asthma sufferers there is a strong possibility of some degree of food allergy as well, and identification of this, by a close watch on symptoms related to the condition, is useful. A food and symptom diary is helpful in this regard, as memory is often unreliable.

Changes in what is eaten

It is useful to eliminate from the diet those factors which are the commonest irritants amongst asthmatics.

These include all dairy produce, chocolate, and eggs. Of course any food might be a factor, but by reforming the diet to avoid the obvious junky-sugary foods (sweets, cakes, colas, etc.) and by avoiding the use of dairy products, including eggs, and chocolate, whilst at the same time trying to include an abundance of fresh vegetables and non-citrus fruit (oranges often produce sensitivity) together with good sources of protein such as chicken or fish (unless there is a proven sensitivity to such a food) the child can be well fed, and out of contact with the main undesirable food factors.

This does not necessarily mean that such foods as are known to cause sensitivity should never be eaten. It is possible for a particular food of this sort to be eaten now and then with no reaction resulting. It is usually the case that an irritant food is likely to become troublesome if consumed two or more times a week by sensitive individuals.

The asthmatic child needs a lot of liquid, so have spring water handy and ensure that no less than 2 ½ , pints daily is consumed (of all liquid) in a child aged 7 to 10. Less liquid would be needed in a younger child.

Use a humidifier in the home, if there is central heating, as very dry air is a potential irritant. Water only should be used in such an appliance. It is also suggested that the child's bedroom should have an air-ionizer in constant use, as should the living room, especially if there are any smokers in the home, or if a TV is in use in that room (see next chapter).

By careful regard to the environment and the diet, and the introduction of aids such as humidifiers and ionizers, much can be done to minimize the dangers, ever-present in the modern home, to the allergic child. It is unlikely that a child could cope with relaxation and visualization exercises without skilful instruction by an expert. However, the general level of stress should be kept down, and fresh air encouraged.

Breathing techniques can be taught to parent and child, and this is a useful contribution to the maintenance of normal function between attacks, and the controlling of the worst aspects of the problem during them.

You're allergic child depends upon your help and guidance, and this approach will support the attempt to achieve control of the condition, whether or not drugs also have to be used to overcome the worst of the symptoms.

11. How ionizers help asthma and hay fever

A small machine called an ionizer can transform the misery of hay fever, and can ease some of the asthmatic's breathing difficulties. An ionizer emits a slight negative electrical charge into the air. If there are particles of pollen, dust, or other pollutants in the air they will be attracted to the negatively charged air molecules (known as ions), where they form a cluster of particles too heavy to remain in the air, and which then fall, leaving the air more desirable to breathe, especially to anyone sensitive to the irritants they contain.

It has long been known that, under certain atmospheric conditions, people feel irritable and out of sorts.

This is when there is a preponderance of positively charged ions in the air. Certain prevailing winds, such as the mistral in France, are also accompanied by such conditions and the incidence of asthma rises dramatically.

If this should be a time of year when pollen is in abundance, then hay fever will be much worse than usual for those susceptible to it.

In contrast, anyone who has breathed deeply of the fresh air after a thunderstorm, or in open countryside, especially near running water, will know what air should be like when it is negatively charged. The ionizing machines now available are small and can if needed be moved from room to room as easily as a portable radio. They produce just the same fresh air feeling as that found in the countryside, even in a polluted city environment.

Offices and work places can be ionized in this way, and a surprising increase in output can often be noted, as people work with more enthusiasm, and there is much less tendency to lethargy, and a lower incidence of infections. The effect is greater where there are elements which are tending to produce the unhealthy positive ionization. These include the presence of machines, central heating, air conditioning, TV sets and computer monitors, artificial fibre carpets, smoke from cigarettes or industrial methods, etc. (The positive ions produced by artificial fibres in carpets and curtains is a factor worth commenting on, as it can be avoided so easily in the homes of individuals with the sort of breathing problems under consideration.)

Research carried out by the University of Surrey showed that more than 70 per cent of individuals using ionizers say that their hay fever has been helped. Also 65 per cent of asthma sufferers say that they achieved some improvement, as did people with chronic bronchitis, when ionizers were used. Some modem offices, when checked for levels of ions, were found to have absolutely no negative ions at all. In nature the healthy ions are created by the rays of the sun (ultra-violet) and ,by natural radiation in the soil and atmosphere. There should naturally be a ratio of about four negative ions to five positive, but in cities this delicate balance can be so disturbed that the ratio can alter to one negative to two positive. It is under such conditions that a malaise and edginess appears in people in general, and aggressive tense feelings occur. In a healthy person this is no more than a minor irritant to life, but to someone with an asthmatic problem it becomes critical.

One of the main helps to hay fever sufferers is the physiological improvement that takes place in the way the hair-like filters called cilia in the nasal passages behave after exposure to negative ionization. When pollution and positive ionization are at work, the cilia become almost stationary and cannot easily move the trapped pollen and dust particles out of the system by their action (together with the normal mucus flow).

Negative ionization restores this function, and helps remove the irritants from the sensitive lining of the breathing passages.

Another effect noted in hay fever sufferers is that negative ions have an actual antihistamine effect.

Large drops in blood histamine levels, of up to 50 per cent, have been noted by researchers, after exposure to negative ionization.

It should be noted that not everyone is helped immediately by the use of ionizers and that about a quarter of those affected by hay fever find only limited relief.

The use of an ionizing machine in the home and/ or workplace is recommended for anyone with hay fever or asthma, for at least a two month trial period. The machines are not very expensive.

12. Some short-term first aid measures

It should be apparent that the measures we have outlined thus far deal, in the main, with the long-term handling of asthma and hay fever, as well as with the underlying changes in the body which have allowed their appearance. Nothing that is advised in this book should preclude the patient from consulting with a doctor regarding the condition, however, and if asthma is present this is probably essential, in case emergency treatment is ever required. The methods outlined base their rationale on the established ability of the body to return to a degree of normality, if the causes of whatever is afflicting it are removed or adequately modified. This is true of all conditions, but not necessarily of all individuals with those conditions.

This is why self-help methods should be seen as preventive and supportive, but not always as curative.

There are aspects of some conditions which require therapeutic intervention, by one type of medical practitioner or another. In asthma the use of osteopathic or chiropractic measures to help to normalize and improve the structural component of the condition is important. This can both help to improve the underlying disturbance affecting the nerve supply to the respiratory organs, and assist in the mechanics of breathing.

The following is a herbal prescription which can be used in an acute asthmatic attack. If it is not effective within two hours the standard medical care should be instituted. It is not suggested that this take the place of emergency care in serious asthma attacks, but that it be kept as a standby for when that may not be available.

Mix equal parts of tinctures of lobelia, capsicum, symphlocarpus and ephedra. Take one teaspoon of this mixture followed by a glass of water every 15 minutes until breathing normalizes.

As stated, if there is no response within a maximum of two hours, medical aid should be sought and standard pharmaceutical intervention instituted.

By incorporating a sound dietary pattern, which has excluded the common 'junk' foods, and also anything which is currently causing symptoms to be produced in terms of allergic reactions, a major contribution to recovery will have been made. Detoxification, as described in Chapter 5, prepares the body for recovery.

The addition of relaxation-meditation exercises, as well as of fresh air and ionization, is a further major step forward.

Supplements

With the detoxified mind and body both relieved of constant stress factors of one sort or another, and with support being given via supplementation to the body's defence mechanisms, a comprehensive programme of long-term value is underway. It is, however, necessary to consider short-term measures which can ease the discomforts and irritations of the symptoms of both asthma and hay fever. These should be seen as supportive, and not to be a comprehensive answer to the overall condition.

No advice is given regarding the use of drugs in these conditions, apart from the notes in Chapter 3, which discuss their actions and side-effects. It can be extremely dangerous to abruptly cease the use of drugs, and any attempt to do so, in the case of an asthmatic, should be under direct guidance from a practitioner who is aware of the history of the individual.

However, nothing that is advised in this section on short-term measures is contraindicated, unless the individual is sensitive, or allergic, to the substances involved, in which case they should obviously be avoided.

Vitamin B12 and asthma

One of the B vitamins cyanocobalamine (B12) has been specifically linked to asthma conditions. Its use in acute stages, and when wheezing is pronounced, has been found to have beneficial results, with no side effects.

This could well relate to the well-known phenomenon of B12 absorption from food being limited in people who have low levels of hydrochloric acid. Thus a programme which increases that factor, as described in Chapter 7, would be expected to improve the levels of B12 automatically.

In therapy, B12 has been used both by injection and by mouth. The results when used intramuscularly seem to be excellent in controlling symptoms, as reported in a number of studies. Doses of 1,000 micrograms by injection were shown to have a greater effect than an enormous 30,000 micrograms (30mg) by mouth, although both methods were satisfactory.

Since most suppliers of oral forms of B12 seldom provide stronger tablets than 500 micrograms, the taking of a dose of 30 milligrams would entail the swallowing of some 60 tablets a day. It would patently be more desirable to improve the body's own ability to absorb B12 from food, and this is what the HCl supplementation, discussed in Chapter 7, is intended to accomplish.

Jonathan Wright recommends attempting another route. It is possible for rapid absorption of some substances to occur from the mouth itself, and he therefore suggests that, in self-treatment, the placing of a dose of 3,000 micrograms under the tongue will lead to absorption and a rapid demonstrable rise in B12levels in the blood (between 90 and 140 per cent increase). However, he points out that this should be compared to a rise of between 500 and 1,000 per cent when B12 is injected. The advice therefore is to try to take B12 by mouth in high doses (either swallowed, or under the tongue until they are dissolved) or to obtain B12 injections from a doctor. If the oral route is effective, well and good, if not, the opportunity exists to discuss the possibility of B12 injections with a medical adviser. It is clear that whilst this approach will often eliminate wheezing it does nothing to eliminate the allergic underlying cause of the problem (which may be related to so many factors, including HCl deficiency). The use of B12 orally, in doses of between 1,000 and 3,000 micrograms daily, should be attempted during attacks and if relief is obtained this should be continued as needed, whilst the underlying conditions which have produced the asthma (stress, diet, allergy, etc.) are dealt with.

The bioflavonoids and asthma

Researchers over the years have discovered a number of chemically similar substances which occur naturally in combination with vitamin C, and which have a specific role in the human economy. They are called bioflavonoids and have at times been called vitamin P.

Their main role appears to be the reduction in permeability of small blood vessels, but more recent research has shown that they enhance vitamin C effects, whatever these might be, and that some of the flavonoids have specific therapeutic functions.

The flavonoids in general have been called 'biological response modifiers', and quercetin is perhaps the most powerful of these. This substance is undoubtedly the most exciting of the flavonoid group and has specific effects in asthma attacks. It is found in the rinds and barks of wild plants and in a number of common foods. It has been shown to inhibit the release, by mast cells in the body, of the substance histamine, when these cells are irritated by allergens.

The release of histamine and other inflammatory mediators from mast cells (and from cells called basophils) is the major factor in the production of the inflammatory response seen in allergies. Mast cells are found in the entire body, but most notably in the blood vessels, respiratory tract, gastrointestinal tract, and skin. It appears that quercetin short circuits the inflammatory response, and in this it can be seen to be acting on the symptoms rather than the cause of the problem.

This means that, in self-help methods, it plays a role which is supportive but not curative. It can safely be used to help when attacks are imminent or current, but

this should only be as part of an overall approach which is trying to normalize the problem. Quercetin also has what is called a 'vitamin C sparing' effect, allowing this invaluable vitamin to function more effectively.

Quercetin thus has a stabilizing effect on irritated mucous membranes. There are other flavonoids which have desirable effects of this sort, such as esculin and umbelliferone - however, quercetin is the most researched and widely available of these useful substances. This is used in a pharmacological manner, which is to say it is used to treat the symptoms of the condition of asthma rather than being seen to be needed to make up a deficiency. There are very few toxic effects reported from the use of quercetin, and doses suggested are of 400 milligrams (mg), three times daily, about twenty minutes before mealtimes.

Excellent common sources of quercetin are onions, dill, bell peppers, elder flowers, witch hazel, pears (peel), apple (peel), Brussels sprouts, kale (which has a content of 50 milligrams of quercetin per kilogram), asparagus, eucalyptus and tarragon.

Vitamin B5 or pantothenic acid (usually marketed as calcium pantothenate) is a specific 'remedy' for many hay fever sufferers. In doses of between 50 and 100mg, taken twice daily, this supports the adrenal glands, and in many individuals appears to reduce the symptoms speedily. Reports from the USA by a number of allergists support this suggestion, and it is worth remembering that vitamin B5 is non-toxic. This can also be useful for asthma sufferers.

In addition, the use of *vitamin* C in large doses has an antihistamine effect, which reduces symptoms appreciably. During hay fever (and asthma) attacks, three doses daily, of between 500 mg and 1000mg of vitamin C, should be taken. If diarrhoea appears then the dose is probably too high, and it should be cut down, but not out. The vitamin C should have bioflavonoids incorporated into it, and this will be stated on the package or label.

Comfrey leaf tea is beneficial in hay fever, especially if coughing is a part of the symptomatology.

The same is true of eating young, tender comfrey leaves. The tea should be made strong, and sweetened with a little honey if needed. Three to five cups a day are usually found to be an adequate quantity. *Nettle tea,* made from the dried young leaves of the plant, is also a useful hay fever aid. Interestingly, nettles contain an abundance of histamine, and it may be that a homoeopathic effect is being achieved by using tea from this plant. The use of *garlic and onions* in abundance is also recommended. If there is a taste for garlic, up to a clove a day can be eaten raw, to good effect. Any odours that linger can be to some extent removed by chewing raw parsley. It is of interest that onions contain an abundance of quercetin, which may account for some of their benefits, although it is thought that the mustard oils which onion contains are more likely to account for the many useful characteristics demonstrated in treating asthma and hay fever.

Brisk exercise is specifically helpful in cases of hay fever, and a few minutes skipping or cycling (static cycle if outdoors is too pollen-rich) has a dramatic effect on the nasal congestion which accompanies the condition.

Asthma first aid includes the use of *vitamin B6* (pyridoxine). This should be taken in doses of between 200mg and 400mg daily, in divided doses. Clinical trials indicate that most asthmatics respond well to this B vitamin, which should be taken together with a vitamin B-complex tablet. Both of these nutrients are available from health food stores. At this level of dosages ofB6 there are no known side-effects, whereas if doses of a level of 2000mg and upwards are taken, some people develop a form of neuritis. The levels suggested are perfectly safe, even for children.

Many *herbal remedies* are recommended for asthmatic conditions. One that seems more effective than others is the herb mullein. Three or four cups of tea a day made from this herb are recommended. It can be obtained from herbalists, or some health stores, or if you can identify it (from a book on herbs) it can be dried at home. The part used is the flower (pick only fresh flowers; once they have turned brown they are of less use). Among the other herbs recommended are henbane, celandine, valerian, and fennel.

Homoeopathic remedies can be helpful in dealing with the underlying traits which predispose towards allergic conditions and in dealing with symptoms.

These would have to be individually assessed and prescribed by a practitioner.

Hydrotherapy

Certain traditional *hydrotherapy* measures are also helpful, and these include the following:

Cold Friction Rub

One of the simplest water treatments. All that is required is a coarse towel and cold water. Dip the towel into cold water and lightly ring it out. Start from the feet, working upwards, and scrub every part of the body with the wet towel. The cold friction should be done quite vigorously, and the final results should show a glowing skin. It may be advisable for beginners to stand with the feet in a bowl of warm water for the first few times. The cold friction rub tones and hardens the skin, prevents chills and bronchitis, and improves the circulation and nervous system.

Baths

The *rising and falling bath* is very easy to carry out at home. The ordinary bath is filled with water at a temperature of 95-100°F (35-38°C). The patient lies in this water, then the hot tap is turned on and the water is allowed to rise to 108-110oF (42-43°C).

Sweating will probably result at this stage and should be maintained for five to six minutes before the temperature is lowered by the addition of cold water to 75-85°F (24-29°C). The object of this bath, like all water treatments, is to dissolve, eliminate and strengthen.

It dissolves poisons into a condition where they can be freely eliminated, assists elimination and strengthens the body. The rising and falling bath should not be taken in cases complicated by heart trouble without expert advice.

The *relaxing* bath is of special benefit to asthma and hay fever subjects, in that it is particularly helpful to 'the nervous system. The temperature of the bath should be kept at about 90-93°F (32-34°C) for as long as forty to sixty minutes. This temperature ensures a pleasant feeling of relaxation, and it is advisable to stay in the water for at least forty minutes to produce the relaxation of nervous tension that is desired. It will often be found that the addition of a little pine oil will make it more effective in asthma cases. It can normally be quite safely taken in all cases, including those with heart trouble, and will be found very beneficial.

The *Epsom salt bath* can quite easily be applied at home. Allow 1 to 1tlb of the commercial Epsom salts for each bath. Epsom salts neutralize the acid waste products of the body and assist the elimination of such acids. It is a particularly useful bath for all cases of asthma and hay fever because of its eliminating effects.

The hot water should not be more than 105°F (40°C), and it is not desirable to stay in the salt bath for more than ten minutes. Over this period there is a danger of palpitation and faintness, especially in elderly people.

It is not advisable to take this bath while fasting, except under supervision, and it is not suitable for heart cases. The salt bath is, however, a very useful addition to home treatment, provided that sensible precautions are observed and the time limit is not exceeded. It is very *necessary* to cool down with a cold splash or shower after a salt bath (as after any hot bath) and to have at least an hour's rest after the treatment. The salt bath should not be taken more than twice in a week.

The *whole foot bath* is extremely useful at a time when an attack of asthma may be pending. Sit with the feet in a bowl of water, as hot as can comfortably be borne. This will draw the blood from the upper parts of the body and reduce the congestion in that area. The same treatment for the hands will often be found effective.

Steaming

Steaming of the nose, throat and chest frequently alleviates the irritated condition of the mucus lining of the air passages and facilitates the expulsion of mucus.

The steam heat penetrates the air-passages more effectively than most forms of heat. While a steam kettle is a useful addition for the home treatment of asthma and hay fever, it is not essential. The ordinary domestic kettle can be made to serve the same purpose.

The kettle should be about two-thirds full of water and a steady jet of steam maintained. The steam must be directed on the nose, throat and chest for at least ten to fifteen minutes, and the process concluded by cold water application to the steamed parts. The addition of a little pine oil to the water used for steaming is advised. It is, of course, possible to steam the head and shoulder regions by bending over a bowl of very hot water while a piece of sheeting covers the head and shoulders and encloses the bowl. This is a very effective method, but it does entail a cramped position which is avoided by the use of a kettle.

Acupuncture and acupressure

Acupuncture has been found to be effective in treating both hay fever and asthma, as have acupressure techniques. Self-help by the use of acupressure requires that the appropriate books on the subject be obtained, and both the methodology and the points themselves learned.

The following are some of the most effective *acupressure* points which can be used as first aid measures to relieve asthma and/ or allergy symptoms.

These are not meant to be substitutes for a comprehensive approach which deals with causes. These methods are meant for symptomatic treatment only.

Seek the points, where they are described, and use direct pressure with a finger or thumb to probe; if they are sensitive to pressure then they are 'active' reflexes, and are suitable for treatment by direct deep pressure for 10 to 20 seconds (enough to cause a 'nice hurt' but not pain). Several should be treated at any one time, one after the other. If symptoms ease during pressure (for example breathing becomes easier, or irritation diminishes) then stop treatment. If no relief is forthcoming then re-examine the location of the point(s)

and ensure that you are on the most sensitive part of the areas. (A 'twinge' should be noted on deep pressure of an active point.) It is also possible that inadequate pressure was used for too short a time.

Trial and error is needed in learning just how hard to press in order to evoke the reflex effect wanted. There are several reflex points involved in any condition. Try various combinations if the hoped-for beneficial response is limited or absent. If no effect is noted, despite correct use of points, then the condition may be too severe to respond to reflex stimulus of this sort.

In any case the response would only be a temporary one unless underlying causes were also being eliminated.

At best expect some hours free of symptoms of allergy, or a marked reduction in symptoms of asthma.

Point 1: This is located on the outer aspect of the elbow and is found by bending the elbow fully and locating the extreme outer edge of the major crease formed by the bend. Mark the point with a finger tip and straighten the elbow before pressing deeply into the tissues. If it is found to be very tender it is active, and can be treated for the symptoms of *hay fever.* One or both sides should be treated in this way. This should be followed by treatment of the next point for best effects.

Point 2: This point is found on the inner thigh about an inch and a half above the level of the top of the knee cap, on a line directly upwards from the prominent inner bone of the ankle. Seek a very tender point here, by deep thumb or finger pressure, and if tender treat it for 10 to 20 seconds, on one or both sides. This is *for hay fever.*

Point 3: This point is found at the level of the elbow crease on the front outer aspect (thumb side). Probe the hollow to the side of the central depression until a very tender point is found, and treat this for 10 to 20 seconds, on one or both sides. This point is suitable for treatment of *asthma or allergic symptoms* such as hay fever. (The previous two points are suitable for hay fever, but not asthma.)

Point 4: This point is found above the major wrist crease on the outer aspect of the back of the forearm, about an inch and a quarter above that crease, in line with the thumbnail. It is in a slight depression above the prominent wrist bone. Seek a tender point by - probing, and when found treat for 10 to 20 seconds by deep pressure, on one or both sides of the body. *This is for treatment of asthma.*

Point 5: This point is on the wrist crease on the front of the forearm, in line with the thumb. Probe for a sensitive point, and treat on one or both sides of the body, for 10 to 20 seconds for *asthma.*

Point 6: This point is found on the back of the forearm about a hand's width above the most prominent wrist crease, in line with the middle finger. Probe for a tender point and treat for 10 to 20 seconds, on one or both sides *for asthma symptoms.*

Point 7: Seek the sensitive points just below the collarbone, in line with the outer margins of the neck, in slight depressions. Treat both sides with deep pressure, for 10 to 20 seconds, for *asthma.*

None of these points should be treated more than twice daily, or the reflexes can become exhausted. If no response is forthcoming from the acupressure therapy, as suggested above, then this method is not for you.

Whether or not these methods assist, it is still necessary to pay attention to the many other methods which can help in dealing with the underlying causes of asthma or hay fever, as described in previous sections.

www.ingramcontent.com/pod-product-compliance
Lightning Source LLC
Chambersburg PA
CBHW070750290526
45795CB00002B/554